Instant

Psychopharmacology

Instant
Psychopharmacology

*Up-to-Date Information about
the Most Commonly Prescribed
Psychiatric Medications*

THIRD EDITION

Ronald J. Diamond, M.D.

W. W. Norton & Company
New York • London

For information about permission to reproduce
selections from this book, write to Permissions,
W. W. Norton & Company, Inc.,
500 Fifth Avenue, New York, NY 10110

For information about special discounts for bulk
purchases, please contact W. W. Norton Special Sales at
specialsales@wwnorton.com or 800-233-4830

Manufacturing by Malloy Printing
Book design by Charlotte Staub
Production manager: Leeann Graham

Library of Congress Cataloging-in-Publication Data

Diamond, Ronald J., 1946–
   Instant psychopharmacology : up-to-date information
about the most commonly prescribed drugs for
emotional health / Ronald J. Diamond. — 3rd ed.
      p. cm.
   Includes bibliographical references and index.
   ISBN 978-0-393-70566-9 (pbk.)
   1. Psychopharmacology—Handbooks, manuals, etc.
2. Psychotropic drugs—Handbooks, manuals, etc.
3. Mental health personnel—Handbooks, manuals, etc.
I. Title.
   RM315.D486 2009
   615'.78—dc22

                                        2008045586

ISBN 13: 978-0-393-70566-9 (pbk.)

W. W. Norton & Company, Inc.,
500 Fifth Avenue, New York, N.Y. 10110
www.wwnorton.com

W. W. Norton & Company Ltd., Castle House,
75/76 Wells Street, London W1T 3QT

1 2 3 4 5 6 7 8 9 0

Contents

Acknowledgments   vii

Preface to the Third Edition   ix

1   The Rules of the Game   1

2   The Basics of Psychopharmacology   19

3   Introduction to Antipsychotic Medications   37

4   Antipsychotic Medications: Medication Profiles   71

5   Antidepressant Medications   114

6   Mood-Stabilizing Medications   155

7   Medications Useful for Anxiety Disorders and
    Sleep Problems   185

8   Miscellaneous Medications   209

9   Medication for People with Borderline
    Personality Disorder   239

Medication List by Generic Name   257

Medication List by Brand Name   262

Medication List by Class   267

Medication List by Cost   270

Bibliography   272

Index   283

Acknowledgments

I have had the joy of working in the same job, at the same place, with some of the same people for more than 30 years. Some of the staff members whom I first met in 1977 are still my colleagues, and some of the consumers I first met in the 1970s are still my patients. We have grown old together over a period of decades. We have married, divorced, had kids, and seen those kids move away. It has given me a perspective that influences how I approach the world.

The Mental Health Center of Dane County in Madison, Wisconsin was my first job out of residency. It is a unique and wonderful place, constantly changing, very much focused on the needs of consumers. As with all bureaucracies and institutions it is not without its flaws, but it remains rooted in values of recovery, cultural competence, and clinical expertise. It is a place that takes the ideas of multidisciplinary teams seriously. It is a place where people from different backgrounds and perspectives really do work together.

I was first hired by my friend and mentor, Dr. Leonard Stein, who, along with Maryanne Test, invented and pioneered the idea of assertive community treatment and changed the face of community psychiatry. I have worked and taught with Dr. Robert Factor and Dr. Fred Coleman for more than 30 years, and the expertise of both are found in this book. My nonmedical colleagues—those with whom I now work and those with whom I have worked over the past 30 years—are way too numerous to list, but they too are part of any wisdom that is in this book. The list includes Dottie Richardson, Bob Mohelinitzky, Tim Otis, Gail Marker, Al Olson, Lynn Brady, Linda Keys, Bill Greer, Karen Stevenson, and many others. It also includes the many consumers who have patiently tried to teach me how to listen, how to be wise, and how to be a better clinician. Along the way they have taught me what medications really do, which is not always the same as what the books say medication is supposed to do.

I want to thank Dr. Jeff Jefferson, psychopharmacologist extraordinaire, and Dr. Alan Rosen, a friend who has been director of a community-based system of care, a humanist, and a practical psychopharmacologist for more than 30 years. Each made notes on the second edition of this book shortly after it was published. These notes have helped to improve this third edition. I want to thank Terri Pelliteri and Pam Valenta for going through drafts of this edition, as they did for the second edition. Dr. Nathan Valentine, a psychiatry resident now at the University of Wisconsin, also read a draft with great care and found errors that I would definitely have missed without his help.

I most want to thank Cher, my wife, for reading the draft, letting me spread out all over the dining room table, feeding me an ongoing supply of chocolate, and in an endless number of other ways being my support. This book is dedicated to her as my life partner, my better half, the person who helps me to be whole.

Preface to the Third Edition

This book started as a handout for a series of lectures on psychopharmacology I first gave in 1974 at the Santa Clara Valley Medical Center in California as a beginning psychiatry resident. At that time, nonphysician staff members, from nurses to social workers to psych techs, were not expected to be educated about medications. Though they spent considerable time sharing their experience and knowledge and had much more contact with the patients than did the physicians, they were discouraged from making suggestions about prescriptions and from monitoring the effects of medications. I began to realize that if these members of the treatment team knew what to look for, they could take on an important role in determining what medication might be useful, how well the medication was working, and what side effects were present. These lectures were my way of sharing information with people who had taught me and conveying my realization that medication decisions needed the input of the entire team of people working with the patient.

As patients have taken increasingly active roles in their own care, they have come to be recognized as clients or, more recently, consumers of mental health care. They, too, must be educated as much as possible. By 1987 I was regularly giving the psychopharmacology lectures for nonmedical staff. One of my own clients found the information extremely useful and asked why clients were not invited. My only response was, I had never thought about it. Since that time, I have invited clients to training sessions I give on psychopharmacology and other topics. At times, this means that state hospital patients leave their inpatient units and go down to the lecture hall. The clients' questions and comments have added to the richness of the teaching, and so far no client has behaved inappropriately during a lecture.

The pace of change in psychopharmacology is accelerating at what feels to be an ever-increasing rate. Now we have new medications introduced yearly, all with very different mechanisms of action. In the old days, the medications within a class were very similar to one another. For example, Navane, Prolixin, Haldol and Stelazine, all traditional antipsychotic medications, all worked the same way, had very similar side effects, and if one did not work the chance of another one working was fairly small. There was little rational reason to use more than one of these medications at a time.

The situation is now very much different. Although medications within a particular class all have somewhat similar mechanisms of action, the differences are much more significant and important than with the older medications. These differences can often be exploited to minimize the impact of side effects. It also means that a given person may respond much better to one of these medications than to another, so switching medications within a class makes much more rational sense than it did when only the older medications were available. Finally, because they have somewhat different mechanisms of action and because we know much more about what these mechanisms are, we can rationally combine medications to increase effectiveness.

This all means that psychopharmacology has become much more complicated as we work to get the maximum benefit from all of the new medications, and maximum benefit from what we now know about how medications work. We are finding that medications can often be useful in treating illnesses beyond those that were listed when the medication was first marketed.

More medications are being used by more people, who are generally staying on them for longer periods of time. Many people are concerned about this trend, and there are books written both pro and con about the philosophical implications of the increased use of psychotropic medications. There are also major financial issues in the increasingly widespread use of very expensive medications. An increasingly portion of health care costs are going to pay for medications that are more effective, safer, better tolerated, more frequently used, and much much more expensive than the medications they replaced.

The premise of this book is that medications will be most useful if the people taking them and the nonmedical clinicians with whom they work know as much as possible about what medications can do to help, and what problems medications can cause. Medication is a tool that can help a person accomplish his or her goals. Before thinking about which medication to use, it is important to be clear what you want the medication to do. Identifying "target symptoms"—clearly defined goals for each medication—allows the client, other clinicians and the prescriber to follow how well a medication is working. It is also critically important to consider medication within the context of the person's life. The focus is not on how to "medicate" a person, but on how a person can use medication. The person taking the medication must be an active participant in the decision and the treatment. Medication alone is almost never enough, but it can help if considered to be a part of the solution rather than *the* solution. This book includes an introduction to the idea of target symptoms, how to integrate medication with other kinds of help, how to balance risk and benefit, and how to improve communication between medical and nonmedical clinicians. These are such important topics that they have been expanded into their own book, *Treatment Collaboration: Improving the Therapist, Prescriber, Client Relationship.*

Despite the hundreds of different medications, psychopharmacology is less complicated than many people believe. Most of the medications used to treat mental illness fall into one of four categories: (1) antipsychotics, (2) antidepressants, (3) mood stabilizers, and (4) antianxiety medications and sleeping pills.

By learning something about each of these four categories of medications, and then learning something about a few variations within each category, you will know much of what you need to know. The book discusses each of these categories, the common medications that are in each category, how they work, what they are used for, and problems that they can cause.

There has been an explosion of new medications. In each category, new medications have replaced the ones that were in common use only a few years ago. These new medications often have advantages over the older medications, but they also come with new problems. The book discusses these new medications, how they work, how they are different from the older medications in each category, the advantages of the newer medications, and the problems that these new medications can cause.

Instant Psychopharmacology is a general introduction. It can be read cover to cover as an overview, or by skipping around, reading the chapters to learn about a particular medication or class of medications. However you use it, this book will increase what you know about medications and allow you to use these medications more effectively. Note that the best way to learn about psychopharmacology is to work with clients; information learned from a book or a lecture can be difficult to remember. The purpose of this book is to give you a sense of the different classes of medications, suggest some basic concepts about medications, and help you build your vocabulary. Your job is to get in the habit of learning about the medications your clients are taking. The way to remember the information in this book is to connect it to a real person. In this, as in many other things, our clients are our best teachers.

During the 12 months prior to publication of this edition, I have been on paid advisory panels for Janssen, maker of Risperdal and Invega, Bristol-Myers Squibb, maker of Abilify, and Pfizer, maker of Geodon. I have given paid talks for Janssen and Bristol-Myers Squibb.

Instant

Psychopharmacology

1

The Rules of the Game

This book is an abridged version of my own views on the use of psychotropic medication. As an increasingly important part of comprehensive mental health treatment, psychotropic medications are used for a wider variety of problems. It is critically important for nonmedical clinicians to know about the medication that their clients are taking as well as to know what medications could be useful that their clients are not yet taking. Nonmedical therapists often know their clients better than the prescribing physician and therefore may be in the best position to help identify target symptoms that would suggest a specific medication. Outside of the client, the nonmedical therapist may also be in the best position to evaluate how well a medication is working.

Medication is often presented as an alternative to other forms of therapy, leading us to believe that we must choose between competing options. The research suggests just the opposite—that appropriately used medication can facilitate other therapy. Conversely, the appropriate use of psychosocial therapy can enhance the effectiveness of medication as well as increase the likelihood that the person will consistently take the medication. This is not to suggest that medications are effective for everyone or that they are not without risks and problems. It does suggest that all therapists, whether philosophically inclined toward biological treatment or not, need to be as knowledgeable as possible about the potential benefits and limitations of psychotropic medications.

This guide is not meant to be definitive. Only those classes of medications I believe are most important are covered, and theoretical issues are largely ignored. *It is essential to keep in mind that the specific indications for use and the specific dosages given are only meant to be rough approximations that fit with my personal experience.* If you are working with a client who is taking a medication with which you are unfamiliar, you can find information about the dosage, contraindications, and side effects in the *Physicians' Desk Reference* (PDR), other recent medication references, or on the Internet.

Although the information in these chapters comes primarily from the references cited at the end of this book, some of it also comes from other papers and books I have read over the years. *Instant Psychopharmacology* is not meant to be an academic treatise, and I have not documented the source for every idea presented.

NINE ESSENTIAL RULES

1. *There are four major classes of medications.* These four classes include the vast majority of psychotropic prescriptions and cover first-line treatment of most common clinical problems. These include:

   - Antipsychotics
   - Antidepressants
   - Mood stabilizers
   - Antianxiety medications and sleeping pills

   I have included a chapter for miscellaneous medications that do not fit into these major classes, but the four major classes constitute the most commonly used medications.

   There are a few different types of medications within each of the above classes. For example, the antidepressant class includes SSRIs (selective serotonin reuptake inhibitors), tricyclics, and MAOIs (monoamine oxidase inhibitors). Medications of the same class tend to be somewhat similar, and medications within the same type are more similar still. Although there are many individual medications, each with its own name and particulars, all you need to know is something about each *class* of medication and the major *types* within each class. If you are familiar with a particular medication, you will already know most of what you need to know about a new or unknown medication of the same type. Learning about a few medications in each class can help you understand the other medications in that class.

2. *All medications have side effects.* All medications exert effects in some part of the body or brain in addition to the specific action that is desired. Some of these effects may be beneficial, some will not help or cause harm, but some are likely to be negative (i.e., they are side effects). All medications have side effects, and all medications have at least some risk. For example, in addition to having anti-pain properties, aspirin decreases the ability of the blood to form clots. Sometimes aspirin is used to decrease blood clotting; other times it is used as a pain reliever. When aspirin is used for pain, its ability to interfere with blood clotting can, on rare occasions, cause very serious problems. Since there are always side effects and risks associated with all medication, a medication should never be used without a clear reason.

3. *Be aware of drug–drug interactions.* Many medications that are very safe alone can cause problems when taken in combination with other drugs. For example, many SSRI antidepressants can interfere with how tricyclic antidepressants are broken down and disposed of by the liver. Giving someone fluoxetine (Prozac [an SSRI antidepressant]) who is also on nortriptyline (a tricyclic antidepressant) can cause a dangerous buildup of the latter. Since fluoxetine stays in the body for a long time, rapidly switching someone from fluoxetine to nortriptyline can have the same effect if it is not done carefully. Furthermore, administering two different drugs that act on different parts of the serotonin system, such as the MAOI tranylcypromine (Parnate) and the SSRI sertraline (Zoloft),

can cause an extremely dangerous serotonergic syndrome (fever, muscle jerking, confusion, rapid fluctuations of blood pressure and other autonomic systems).

4. *Ask about other medications.* Always ask about *all* other medications the person is taking, both prescription and nonprescription, including herbal supplements and vitamins. Many medications used to control high blood pressure, for example, can cause or exacerbate depression. Changing an offending medication may be much more effective than adding another medication. Often people will not mention herbal remedies or birth control pills unless they are specifically asked.

5. *Ask about other medical problems.* Ask about any medical problems the person is currently experiencing or has had in the past. We are in the business of treating the "whole person," and it is important to realize the extent to which medical illness and nonpsychiatric medications can influence mood and behavior.

6. *The use of psychiatric medication during pregnancy presents a difficult dilemma.* It is never possible to say that any medication taken by a pregnant woman is 100% safe for the fetus. Researchers can study the effect of a medication on a pregnant animal. They can also look at the rate of birth defects in children whose mothers took a particular medication and compare this rate to the risk of birth defects in children of women with similar health problems whose mothers did not take the medication. A researcher can say only that so far, an effect on the fetus has not been found. This suggests that if there is a problem, it is likely to be either *not obvious* or *not frequent.* The risk of birth defects is known to be significant when a pregnant woman is taking some drugs, such as alcohol, and some medications, such as valproic acid (Depakote) or carbamazepine (Tegretol). Many other medications have risks that are more complicated to assess. Although some risk may be found as more research is done, available data have not demonstrated that antidepressant medications are dangerous to the developing fetus, with the exception of paroxetine

(Paxil). However, newborns of mothers who are taking an antidepressant medication may experience some withdrawal problems at birth. As with every medication decision, there must be a balance of risks and benefits; after all, there can be negative effects on the developing fetus when the mother is severely depressed or psychotic. Medication can potentially help as well as hurt. A woman who becomes pregnant or is thinking of becoming pregnant should discuss the specific risks with her physician and get as much up-to-date information as possible.

7. *Ask about medication allergies.* Be aware that people can have allergic reactions to any medication. Ask the client about medication allergies *before* any medication is prescribed.

8. *Be careful not to confuse different medications that have very similar names.* Different medications often have very similar names. For example, clonazepam (Klonopin) is a benzodiazepine with anticonvulsant properties; clonidine (Catapres) is an antihypertensive medication often used to help decrease the symptoms of narcotic and other drug withdrawal; clozapine (Clozaril) is a new antipsychotic medication; and clomipramine (Anafranil) is an antidepressant medication that is effective in obsessive–compulsive disorder. Every medication has a generic name as well as a brand name from each manufacturer. A particular medication will always have only one generic name, but if it is made by several pharmaceutical companies, each company will give the medication a different trade name. For example, desipramine is the generic name for a common antidepressant that is marketed by one company under the name Norpramin and by another company under the name Pertofrane. The *PDR* is a common reference that cross-lists generic and trade names for all prescription medications.

9. *No one knows everything.* The most important thing is to recognize what you do not know, and how to get help. At some point, everyone calls someone else for help. A nonmedical clinician may get help from a psychiatrist; a psychiatrist may refer to an expert psychopharmacologist. For more informa-

tion about medication, refer to the resources listed in the bibliography.

THOUGHTS ON THE CLIENT/CLINICIAN/ PSYCHIATRIST RELATIONSHIP

The client, clinician, and psychiatrist must operate as a team, and to a large extent medication decisions should be made jointly by those team members. The client's support system, including family members, can also be an important part of the team. The functioning of this team and the roles of each of the team members is the topic of an entire book (Diamond & Schaeffler, 2007).

The purpose of any medication should be to help the person taking it feel better, function better, and be more in control of his or her own life. Medication is a tool that the person can use in his or her own recovery process, but only if the person is informed about medication issues and involved in medication decisions. The nonmedical clinician typically spends much more time with the client, knows the client better, and knows more about how the client is functioning and feeling than does the psychiatrist. The more the clinician knows about what to expect from medications, how they might help, and what side effects to look for, the more he or she will be able to help educate and involve the client and make sure that the psychiatrist has the information needed to make an informed decision about medication. Specific target goals for what it is hoped a medication will accomplish cannot be developed in isolation.

The psychiatrist has ultimate authority over which medication will be prescribed. In most cases, the client has ultimate authority over what medication he or she will decide to take. The nonmedical clinician has the most information, next to the psychiatrist, about how medication can be most useful and, next to the client him- or herself, the clearest sense of whether it has worked in that particular client. Everyone on the team must be aware of the concerns and goals of the other team members. My strong preference is that medication assessments be made with the psychiatrist, nonmedical clinician, and client all participating in the assessment and sharing information with each other.

Often a number of medication options may seem fairly reasonable. The questions that arise should include medication "A" or "B" be started, should the dose be 10 mg or 15 mg, should the medication be started today or should more time be allowed to see what is happening without medication or before changing medication? If there is not a really good reason to choose one option over the other, the client should be allowed to decide. It is, after all, the client's life. I often say that I, as the prescriber, get a vote, the case manager gets a vote, the client's family gets a vote, and the client gets 10 votes.

It is important to think about when and how much information should be shared. When working with a very anxious, frightened, or confused person who is not processing information well, focus on the information needed to make immediate decisions. Giving too much information all at once to someone who is very upset can overload him or her and actually get in the way of learning. Basic information about how the medication might help, ways for both clients and clinicians to determine if the medication is working, and common side effects should be discussed even with an acutely upset person.

Over time, the prescriber should initiate a more in-depth discussion of the risks and benefits, long-term side effects, and other issues about the medication so that the client can be an informed collaborator in his or her own treatment. Printed medication information sheets, written at an appropriate reading level, are very useful. All of us will absorb less information when we are anxious, and people are very often anxious during a psychiatric assessment. Repeating the same information in subsequent visits is often necessary for people to be able to remember and understand complicated issues.

Withholding information about side effects or alternative treatments is paternalistic and disrespectful; moreover, it interferes with the long-term relationship building that promotes effective treatment and helps the client make responsible decisions about his or her medication. Prescribers often fear that too much information about side effects may discourage a person from taking medication. My experience is that a frank, open, balanced discussion that includes a clear explanation of both risks and benefits promotes long-term medication use. I use my own judgment to decide how quickly and how much information I should share, but my assumption is that over time I will provide as much information as possible. Some clinicians worry that clients will stop taking a medication if they are given too much information about possible side effects. If a person is determined to stop taking medication, information on side effects and benefits is unlikely to sway him or her one way or the other. In any case, sharing information in a straightforward way promotes a healthy relationship that is essential for regular medication use.

COMMUNICATING WITH PHYSICIANS

Nonmedical mental health professionals, such as social workers, have learned to communicate very differently than have physicians. Training for social work stresses knowing all aspects of the client's situation. When social workers talk with one another, they illustrate their competence by demonstrating that they know their clients very well. Their clinical descriptions tend to be rich in detail. Physicians, on the other hand, are trained to focus on just the data that are needed to quickly make a decision. When physicians talk with each other about a patient, they present a very tightly focused summary of the patient and the problem and leave out all information that is not directly relevant to the decision at hand. There tends to be little value on information that might allow the physician to understand the person better, unless this would directly help the decision that needs to be made *now*. This communication style is reinforced by the limited amount of time available for physicians to talk with each other.

Nonmedical staff often pass on information at treatment planning meetings or team meetings where there is at least some time set aside to talk about clients. Physicians, including psychiatrists, often find themselves talking about a client in the brief gaps between patient visits, when there are only a few minutes to answer a phone call or write a note. Given these time constraints, the physician has learned to get to the point quickly.

Social workers often feel that the physician's ultra-brief data-based communication style reflects someone who is cold, disinterested, and does not really know the client very well. Physicians, on the other hand, see the social worker's detailed descriptions as long, rambling, disorganized discussions that never really address the immediate problem. This is not an issue of one profession being right and the other wrong, but rather professional and cultural differences in socialization and communication style.

Understanding these differences can help make communication easier. If a social worker wants to effectively communicate with a physician, he or she should try to organize the point being made, leave out extra details, and be aware of any time limitations. If a physician wants to communicate with a social worker, he or she should use a less abbreviated style and value the richness of detail provided by the social worker.

THOUGHTS FOR THE PERSON WHO IS TAKING MEDICATION

Medications are a tool that can help you cope with mental illness. Modern medications are extremely effective in helping people live with many different kinds of mental illness, from anxiety disorders to depression to schizophrenia. Medications do not always work as well as we might hope, and they often have more side effects than we would like. Some people have a goal to take as little medication as possible or to get off medication as soon as possible. I personally feel that a better goal is to figure out how to use medication so that you can live a life as close as possible to the one you would like.

I talk with many clients who tell me that they have already tried many medications, and that medications do not work for them. They have essentially given up on trying medications, even though their life continues to be very different than they might like, and even though they are bothered by symptoms that get in their way. If medications are tools, and if the first one does not work, it is important to try as many tools as possible before giving up. If a person has symptoms that might respond to a medication, and if those symptoms are getting in the way of living a full life, then I continue to encourage the person to try different medications until we find one that does the job.

I think it is very important for anyone taking medications to get as much information about them as possible. Gathering ample information can help you figure out what else you might want to ask your psychiatrist. It can also help you to understand what kinds of side effects you might experience and to be realistic about how your medications can help. Finally, having more information can help you make better decisions about whether you are willing to take the medications prescribed by your psychiatrist.

Clients often have many questions about their medication that they never ask. Sometimes they find it difficult to ask their psychiatrist questions, or there is not enough time to ask questions, or they feel intimidated, or they do not know how to put their questions into words. It is often helpful to write down questions so that you can remember them. Others find it helpful to practice, with a friend or therapist, what they want to say to the psychiatrist. Appointments with psychiatrists are often shorter than either you or the psychiatrist would like. It may not be possible to get all questions answered in one visit. Think about which questions are most important and which can be put off until your next visit.

The following ideas are important if you are going to be involved in making decisions about your own medication.

1. *Make sure that you know what medication you are taking.*
   Ask the psychiatrist or nurse to write down the name of each

medication, along with instructions about how you are supposed to take it.

2. *Make sure you know what each medication is supposed to do.* What symptoms is each supposed to help? How will you know if it is helping? How long will it take to know if the medication is helping?

3. Many different kinds of symptoms can be helped by medication. What kinds of symptoms do you have? *How much do these symptoms interfere with things you want to do?* Are your symptoms interfering with having friends, getting a job, going shopping, enjoying things?

4. *Besides taking medication, what other things can you do to control your symptoms?* What have you tried? What has worked and what has not? Often there are lots of things that you can do to control symptoms and achieve your own goals. Medication may be an important part of this overall plan, but it will work better if it is combined with other ways of controlling symptoms.

5. *Work with your prescriber and other clinicians to develop your own list of goals*, and then track whether the medication helps you achieve them. Are you better able to go shopping, talk to people, or read a book since you began taking the medication? Involve your psychiatrist in your goals. What do you want from your medication?

6. *Make sure that your prescriber is aware of anything that you feel could be a medication side effect.* Some side effects, such as the restlessness that some people feel with antipsychotic medication, are extremely difficult to tolerate. Other side effects, such as the sexual problems caused by a number of antipsychotic and antidepressant medications, may be embarrassing to talk about. Your psychiatrist cannot help with these side effects if he or she is not aware of them.

There are more and more ways for clients to become educated about their medication. There are many books about medication that are easy to understand. There is information on the Internet about medication, some from sites that are reliable and some less reliable. There is also a growing number of what are called "decision aids"—tools that help clients make medication decisions. Some of these are just information sheets handed out with medication, but a growing number of decision aids actually help people think through their choices. Some are paper-based, and some use a computer to help a client make a medication decision. These decision aids provide a structure that can help clients to think about what they want medication to do and then think about how well their current medication is doing this. The best of these decision aids help clients think about all of their options and the consequences of each decision (Deegan et al.). This kind of structured thinking can help a client to become more of a real participant in the decisions that are affecting his or her life.

THOUGHTS FOR NONMEDICAL CLINICIANS: COMPLIANCE AND COLLABORATION

Most people with chronic illness do not take their medication as prescribed by their doctor. This is equally true for people with chronic medical illness as it is for people with chronic mental illness. Not taking medication as prescribed is often addressed as a problem with medication "compliance." The word *compliance* assumes that the client should comply or follow the prescription of the physician. Ideally, the client–clinician relationship is a collaborative one. The goal is to work *with* the person so that he or she takes the medication in a way that maximizes its effectiveness and minimizes its side effects—which typically means taking medication regularly. This issue of compliance and collaboration deserves an entire book, but there are a few short hints that can be used.

1. *Work to understand the person's view about his or her problem and beliefs about medication.* We are unlikely to take a medication for a problem that we do not feel is fixable, or if

we are convinced that medication is unlikely to be helpful. Our beliefs about the nature of a problem will influence the kinds of help any of us would be willing to accept, including what kinds of medication we are willing to take.

2. *Simplify the medication-taking routine.* The more bottles that must be opened and the more times of day that medication must be taken, the less likely it is that the medication will be taken reliably. People are fairly reliable about taking a medication once a day. It is more difficult for most people to take medication twice a day, and almost impossible for most people to take medication reliably three or four times a day. Most medications used in psychiatry, including lithium and antipsychotics, can be taken once a day. Work with the physician to simplify the medication regime whenever possible.

3. *Suggest that the client take the medication along with some other regular activity.* Taking medication with breakfast or when brushing one's teeth makes it easier to remember.

4. *Arrange packaging* that helps remind the person to take his or her medication. Plastic containers that allow the person to load a week's worth of medication into compartments labeled by the day of the week can help. At times we have made arrangements with our local pharmacy to package medication in individual plastic envelopes, one for each time a medication should be taken. For example, a person taking four different medications simply takes the medication in the "Monday morning" envelope. This method eliminates the need to keep track of different pills from different pill bottles.

5. *Pay attention to side effects.* Take the person's reports of side effects seriously. Even subtle side effects that are unrecognized and untreated can lead a person to decide to discontinue medication. Akathisia, the motor restlessness that comes from some antipsychotic medications and, on rare occasions, from some antidepressants, is extremely uncomfortable, and people often stop taking medication because of it. Many side effects, including akathisia, that are not visible to others can be a problem for the person taking the medication. For exam-

ple, people with akathisia may feel very uncomfortable even if they do not outwardly show the motor restlessness that is commonly part of the side effect.

6. *Be interested in the person's medication use.* Ask what medications the person is taking. If a client decides to take more or less medication, ask how he or she made that decision. View changes the person has made in medication use as the beginning of a conversation, rather than as an indication that the person has done something wrong. Most client-initiated medication changes are not just accidents or figments of some psychotic process. To be useful, we must understand the client's decision-making process.

7. *Connect the medication in concrete ways to the person's own life goals.* If getting a job is what the person wants most then, he or she is going to be more willing to take medication if he or she believes that taking the medication really will help secure a job. Moreover, the person is likely to keep taking the medication if he or she actually gets a job. Continued medication use is often associated with clinical follow-through: clinicians keep the promises of assistance that they have made to clients.

8. *Arrange for medication to be supervised* when necessary. A person who is willing but regularly forgets to take medication can be helped by regular phone calls, by visits from a friend or family member, or from a clinician if mobile outreach services are available.

BEFORE STARTING ANY MEDICATION

1. *A diagnosis needs to be made first.* Medications should not be given just because a person is upset or even in response to symptoms of psychosis. First it is necessary to become clear about the entire situation.

   Corollary A: Delirium needs to be ruled out first. Delirium is easily confused with psychosis but can be distinguished by a careful mental status exam. People with delirium are often disoriented and almost always have memory impairment.

Corollary B: Medical illness or drug intoxication needs to be considered, as they may present as psychosis.

2. *A medication history needs to be obtained* (what medications the person has taken in the past, in what doses, with what effects). If a person previously has had a good response to a particular medication, it makes sense to restart that same drug.

3. *Follow treatment by picking out specific target symptoms and target goals.* Auditory hallucinations might be a target symptom for one person, disorganized thinking for another person, and social withdrawal for yet another. Functional goals are also extremely useful in helping connect medication to real-life changes. Monitoring a person's ability to get out of his or her apartment more often, or to read, or to go grocery shopping may be a very useful way of understanding what kind of impact the medication is having on the person's life. *Write these goals down and make sure that everyone has a copy.* Having a written list of goals for each medication can be very useful for the client and the other members of the team.

AFTER STARTING A MEDICATION

1. *Medications should be adjusted according to target symptoms and side effects.*

2. *More is not necessarily better.* Too much of most medications can cause an increase in side effects without necessarily being any more effective. Side effects can make the person's clinical symptoms worse, and at times drug side effects are difficult to distinguish from the illness being treated. At the same time, too low a dose of medication can prolong discomfort and disability. Most medications take days or weeks to have any effect. Some medications need to be started at a low dose and then increased to an effective dose. Other medications can be started at a dose that is typically effective, and increasing them too soon can lead to too much medication being prescribed. These are all issues that should be discussed with the physician *before* initiating the medication.

3. *Actively look for side effects.* Many medications cause some degree of discomfort. Make sure that the person knows about possible side effects before starting a new medication. Actively monitoring and treating side effects will help people feel more comfortable and will also increase their willingness to continue taking the medications.

Some Thoughts on Side Effects

As already discussed, all medications have side effects. The side effects mentioned in this and other books are those that are most common, experienced by most people taking the medication. People are not the same, and not all people respond or react to the medications in the same way. Some people have side effects that are not listed in the books, or side effects that the prescribing physician has not heard reported before. All reported side effects should be taken seriously. Some may turn out to be unrelated to the medication, whereas others may be related to medication even if they are not on the list of well-known problems. All are part of the experience of the person taking the medication and need to be addressed.

If Medication Does Not Work

The medications used in psychiatry are generally as effective as any of the medications used in the rest of medicine. An antidepressant is as likely to help someone who is suffering from major depression as an antibiotic is to help someone with pneumonia. No medication in any field of medicine works 100% of the time.

As with many of the medications used in physical illness, psychiatric medications control symptoms, relieve pain, and preserve function, but they do not cure the underlying condition. This can be frustrating, but it is common with most psychiatric as well as nonpsychiatric medications.

If medication does not work, consider the following questions:

1. *Is the diagnosis correct?* Treatment is unlikely to work if the wrong illness is being treated. Correcting someone's biological predisposition to depression is less likely to be effective if the person is being overwhelmed by social stressors.
2. *Has a medical illness gone unrecognized?* The most conservative estimate is that 10% of psychiatric patients have unrecognized medical illnesses that are causing or contributing to their mental disorder.
3. *Is substance abuse interfering?* All of the common psychiatric symptoms can be caused, or made worse, by alcohol, stimulants, or other drugs.
4. *Is the person taking the medication?* Estimates are that half of all patients do not take medications as prescribed. A medication is unlikely to work if it is not being taken, or not being taken correctly.
5. *Has the dose been high enough for a long enough period of time?* Almost all of the medications used in psychiatry take days to weeks to be effective. Some medications, such as clozapine, can take months. Too often people quit taking the medication before it has had a chance to work. Many clients who are labeled "nonresponders" go from one medication to another without giving any of them enough time to see if they would be effective. In other cases, a person will have stayed on a medication long enough but at such a low dose that it is unlikely to help.
5. *Are there stressors in the person's life that would interfere with the medication's efficacy?* Medications do not work by themselves. Too often, people with mental illness deal with poor housing, not enough money, and disrupted social support systems. Although medication is important, it is only one part of the treatment process.
7. *Are there other things that the person can do, in addition to taking the medication, to promote his or her own recovery?* Almost all clients are doing the best that they can; their ill-

ness is not their fault. At the same time, if their life is going to change, they are going to have to be involved in making the change happen. What makes the symptoms better? What makes them worse? Are there behavioral strategies or activities that can help ameliorate some of the symptoms? A critical part of collaboration is encouraging the client to be an active partner in his or her own treatment. Medication is not the only treatment that works. Cognitive–behavioral therapy, skill training, interpersonal psychotherapy, and other strategies can all help people with various kinds of mental illness to improve their quality of life.

2

The Basics of Psychopharmacology

It is increasingly difficult to provide a simple classification of psychotropic medications. These medications are commonly associated with the initial use described for them. Many, if not most, of the medications on this list have other uses that are often as important as this original indication. For example, SSRI antidepressants are also very effective antianxiety, anti-panic, and anti-obsessional medication, yet we still call them antidepressants. They could just as easily have been introduced as antianxiety and anti-panic medications, and their use as antidepressants could have been discovered later. Several of the antidepressants seem to be very useful in chronic pain conditions, even for people who are not depressed. The second-generation antipsychotic medications all have excellent efficacy as a mood stabilizer, even for people who have no psychotic symptoms. Lithium is effective for certain kinds of "hair-trigger" anger outbursts, even if the person has no hint of bipolar disorder.

Some of these uses for a medication have a formal FDA (U.S. Food and Drug Administration) indication. An FDA indication requires that the company that makes the medication formally request the FDA to list this new use of the medication. This process requires research that is specifically focused on this new use and typically costs millions of dollars. Pharmaceutical companies are willing to make this investment for expensive medications that will have patent protection for years to come, but they are generally not willing to make this investment for medications that are now available, or about to be available, as a less expensive generic. For example, there is strong research support that carbamazepine is an effective mood stabilizer, and it is widely used in Europe for this purpose. Because it is available as generic, no U.S. pharmaceutical company went to the expense of getting an FDA indication for carbamazepine as a mood stabilizer until a longer acting form that could be patented was available. Not having an FDA indication for a particular disorder does not keep that medication from being prescribed for that disorder, but it does mean that there has been no formal review by the FDA for the research support for that use.

The classification of medications given below is for the initial use of each of these medications. This brief list does not give a full description of all the ways these medications are now used. Medications marked with an asterisk are available as a long-acting injection as well as tablets or capsules.

  I. Antipsychotic Medications
    A. *Second-generation antipsychotic medications* used to be called *atypical*, but since these are now accepted as first-line treatment, they are no longer "atypical." These antipsychotic medications have much less likelihood of causing motor side effects. Although these medications are classified as "antipsychotics," they are all effective mood stabilizers, even for people who are not psychotic:
       1. clozapine (Clozaril)
       2. risperidone (Risperdal)*
       3. olanzapine (Zyprexa)
       4. quetiapine (Seroquel)
       5. ziprasidone (Geodon)
       6. aripirazole (Abilify)
       7. paliperidone (Invega)*
    B. *First-generation antipsychotic medications* are sometimes referred to as *neuroleptics*. The newer second-generation antipsychotic medications are now much more commonly used than the older first-generation medications, but research suggests that the second-

generation medications may not always be more effective or always have fewer side effects. Some of the more common first-generation antipsychotics:

1. phenothiazines
   a. most sedating; e.g., chlorpromazine (Thorazine),
   b. intermediate sedating; e.g. perphenazine (Trilafon)
   c. least sedating; e.g., fluphenazine (Prolixin)*
2. butyrophenomes; e.g., haloperidol (Haldol)*
3. thioxanthenes; e.g., thiothixene (Navane)
4. Miscellaneous traditional neuroleptics:
   a. molindone (Moban)
   b. loxapine (Loxitane)

II. Antidepressants

Although these medications are labeled *antidepressants*, many of them also have significant antianxiety, anti-panic, and anti-obsession properties. Some are also very helpful with chronic pain conditions, even for people who are not depressed.

A. Serotonin/norepinephrine antidepressants:
   1. Selective serotonin and norepinephrine reuptake blockers
      a. Selective serotonin reuptake inhibitors (SSRIs); e.g., fluoxetine (Prozac), sertraline (Zoloft)
      b. Selective serotonin and noradrenergic reuptake blockers; e.g., venlafaxine (Effexor), duloxetine (Cymbalta)
      c. Selective noradrenergic reuptake blockers; e.g., reboxetine (not available in the U.S.)
   2. Alpha-2 antagonist; e.g., mirtazapine (Remeron)
   3. Serotonin 2a receptor blockers; e.g., nefazodone (Serzone), trazodone (Desyrel)
B. Norepinephrine and dopamine reuptake blockers; e.g., bupropion (Wellbutrin)
C. Tricyclic antidepressants:
   1. Norepinephrine reuptake blockade: e.g., desipramine (Norpramin), amitriptyline (Elavil)

    2. Serotonin reuptake blockade; e.g., Clomipramine (Anafranil)

D. Monoamine oxidase inhibitors (MAOIs):
    1. Pills or capsules; e.g., phenelzine (Nardil), tranylcypromine (Parnate)
    2. Skin patch (fewer interactions with food; e.g., selegiline transdermal patch [Emsam])

III. Mood Stabilizers

A. Lithium (Eskalith, Lithobid)

B. Anticonvulsants with mood-stabilizing properties:
    1. carbamazepine (Tegretol)
    2. oxcarbazepine (Trileptal; active metabolite of carbamazepine with fewer side effects)
    2. Valproic acid (Depakene), divalproex sodium (Depakote)
    3. lamotrigine (Lamictal)

C. Anticonvulsants that may be useful for other conditions but have no clear mood-stabilizing properties: e.g., gabapentin (Neurontin), topiramate (Topamax), pregabalin (Lyrica)

IV. Antianxiety Medications and Sleeping Pills

A. Medications useful for both sleep and anxiety:
    1. Benzodiazepines marketed as anxiolytics; e.g., diazepam (Valium) and lorazepam (Ativan)
    2. Benzodiazepines marketed as sleeping pills; e.g., flurazepam (Dalmane) and temazepam (Restoril)

B. Medications useful for anxiety, not effective for sleep:
    1. buspirone (Buspar)
    2. SSRI and SNRI antidepressants are also effective in treatment of anxiety

C. Sleeping medications, not as helpful for anxiety:
    1. Selective GABAA agonists, e.g., zolpidem (Ambien) and zaleplon (Sonata)
    3. Melatonin receptor agonists: e.g., ramelteon (Rozerem)
    4. trazodone (Desyrel; sedative antidepressant)

  5. Sedative antihistamines; e.g., diphenhydramine (Benadryl)
V. Miscellaneous
  A. Beta-blockers—e.g., propranolol (Inderal), atenolol (Tenormin)—are helpful in a variety of situations, including performance anxiety and akathisia (motor restlessness as a side effect of antipsychotic medication).
  B. Medications for ADHD:
    1. stimulants; e.g., methylphenidate (Ritalin), amphetamine (Dexedrine)
    2. Nonstimulant: atomoxetine (Strattera)
  C. Medications for PTSD:
    1. Alpha-2 adrenergic agonist; e.g., clonidine (Catapres), guanfacine (Tenex)
    2. Alpha-1 adrenergic antagonist; e.g., prazosin (Minipress)
  D. Medications to help manage substance abuse and dependence:
    1. Medications to help manage alcohol abuse
      a disulfiram (Antabuse)
      b. naltrexone (ReVia)
      c. acamprosate (Campral)
    2. Medications to help manage opiate dependence
      a. methadone
      b. buprenorphine (Suboxone)
    3. Medications to help manage smoking cessation
      a. varenicline (Chantix)
      b. bupropion (Zyban, Wellbutrin)
      c. Nicotine replacement
  D. Antiparkinsonian medications (decrease extrapyramidal side effects):
    1. Anticholinergic; e.g., benztropine (Cogentin), diphenhydramine (Benadryl)
    2. Dopaminergic; e.g., amantadine (Symmetrel)
  E. Cognitive enhancers (for use in dementia)
    1. Cholinergic medications; e.g., donepezil (Aricept)
    2. MNDA receptor antagonist: memantine (Namenda)

How Do Medications Work?

Most psychotropic drugs affect the brain by increasing or decreasing the activity of various *neurotransmitters,* which are chemical messengers that operate between adjacent nerve cells. The space between two nerve cells is called a *synapse.* Neurotransmitters are released from a nerve cell into the synapse, and they travel across the synapse to act on the receptors of the next nerve cell.

Some neurotransmitters are *excitatory* and trigger the firing of the nerve cell. Other neurotransmitters are *inhibitory* and inhibit the firing of the cell. Receptors can also be either presynaptic or postsynaptic. Presynaptic receptors are on the nerve cell that is releasing the neurotransmitter and act as a brake or feedback mechanism controlling the amount of neurotransmitter released. Postsynaptic receptors are on the receiving side of the synapse. Different medications work by either excitatory or inhibitory action at the presynaptic or postsynaptic receptors, or in somewhat complicated combinations of these.

Each neurotransmitter operates in multiple places in the brain, causing many different effects. More than 50 neurotransmitters have been identified. The important ones in psychopharmacology are *acetylcholine, dopamine, adrenaline* (or *epinephrine*), *noradrenaline* (or *norepinephrine*), *serotonin,* and *GABA* (*gamma-aminobutyric acid*). A number of new neurotransmitters are beginning to be discussed in the literature and medications are currently being developed that affect glutamate, glycine, nicotinic acid, melatonin, substance P receptors, and many others.

A particular kind of nerve cell typically releases only one kind of neurotransmitter. A serotonin cell, for example, releases only serotonin, and a dopamine cell releases only dopamine. Each cell has receptors for many different neurotransmitters. A single nerve cell may have receptors for dopamine, serotonin, glutamate, acetylcholine, and more. Even more complicated, each neurotransmitter affects a number of different receptors. There are at least five different dopamine receptors (labeled D_1, D_2, and so on), and there are at least 15 different serotonin receptors, with more being discovered all the time. Each of these different receptors has different actions in the brain and different responses to medications.

A medication that affects a receptor can either block that receptor, thereby decreasing its activity, or directly stimulate that receptor and increase its firing. *Agonists* are chemicals or medications that stimulate a specific receptor. *Antagonists* are medications that block the action of a neurotransmitter. For example, dopamine is an agonist for dopamine receptors; it stimulates the activity of those receptors. Haloperidol is an antagonist that blocks the action of dopamine, at least at the D_2 receptor. It is, of course, more complicated than this statement belies. A medication, such as aripiprazole (Abilify) is a *partial* agonist and thus work as both an antagonist that blocks the receptor and also weakly as an agonist that stimulates the receptor so that it fires at some set rate less than it would if the actual neurotransmitter were stimulating it. The same medication can stimulate some receptors and block others.

NEUROTRANSMITTERS OF INTEREST IN MENTAL ILLNESS

Acetylcholine

The neurotransmitter acetylcholine is widely present throughout the body. Acetylcholine receptors are called *cholinergic* receptors (choline = cholinergic), and medications that block the action of acetylcholine by blocking receptors are called *anticholinergic*. Many commonly used medications have some anticholinergic properties. Anticholinergic medications are most commonly used in psychiatry to treat some of the motor side effects associated with first-generation antipsychotics. There are two kinds of receptors that respond to acetylcholine. These are called *muscarinic*, and *nicotinic* receptors, each with its own subsets, so that there are actually five different muscarinic receptors and a growing number of identified nicotinic receptors.

Cholinergic muscarinic receptors control such areas as salivation, gut motility, and the lens in the eye, as well as thinking and memory. Therefore, medications that block the cholinergic system typically cause dry mouth, blurred vision, constipation, problems with memory, and, in some cases, delirium. Decreased activity at the M_1 (muscarinic) receptor appears to be associated with cognitive dysfunction in schizophrenia, and it is expected that a number of medications will be developed in an attempt to increase M_1 activity.

Cholinergic nicotinic receptors (called *nicotinic* because they are extremely sensitive to nicotine) may affect thinking and "gating," which is the ability to screen out extraneous information. One theory about schizophrenia is that the illness causes problems in gating information, therefore too much information is sent to the cortex. A very high percentage of people with schizophrenia smoke; these people may be using the nicotine in cigarettes in a "naturalistic" attempt to overcome this gating problem.

Medications that increase cholinergic activity in the brain are "cognitive enhancers" and are being used for the symptomatic treatment of dementia, and perhaps to reverse some of the cognitive deficits caused by schizophrenia.

Dopamine

Dopamine is associated with psychosis, focused attention, addiction, and drugs of abuse. A number of different dopamine receptors have been identified. Traditional antipsychotic medications block the action of dopamine at the receptor sites in the receiving cells. Specifically, they block what are called D_2 receptors. Any drug, such as cocaine, that increases D_2 activity can cause psychotic symptoms. Any medication that blocks D_2 receptors, specifically in the mesolimbic part of the brain, is an antipsychotic. The blocking of dopamine receptors in other parts of the brain causes many of the side effects of antipsychotic medications.

The second-generation or atypical antipsychotic medications are much more selective; they tend to block just the receptors needed to treat positive symptoms, such as hallucinations and delusions, while having much less effect on other dopamine receptors. This selectivity produces fewer side effects.

Epinephrine

As noted, another name for adrenaline is *epinephrine*. There are two kinds of adrenergic receptors: alpha and beta. Beta-blockers (propranolol) block the beta set of these receptors, leaving the alpha set intact. Peripherally, outside of the brain, epinephrine has a wide variety of effects, including increasing heart rate and blood pressure. In the brain it is involved in maintaining focus, decreasing depression, and feeling pleasure.

GABA

GABA inhibits or decreases the activity of nerve cells. It is found throughout the brain and is the *primary inhibitory neurotransmitter*. Antianxiety medications such as diazepam (Valium) and sleep medications such as zolpidem (Ambien) both make GABA work more effectively. That is, diazepam alone does not inhibit nerve cell activity, but diazepam + GABA inhibit the firing of the cell more than just GABA alone. This means that GABA continues to control how much inhibition occurs. Benzodiazepines are much safer than older medications such as Seconal (or alcohol), which directly inhibit brain activity to the point where people can stop breathing. Zolpidem and diazepam work at slightly different places in the GABA receptor, causing one (Zolpidem) to have more antianxiety effect and the other (diazepam) more effect on sleep.

Glutamate

Glutamate stimulates the firing of nerve cells. It is present in large amounts throughout the brain and is the *primary excitatory neurotransmitter*. Glutamate is essential for normal brain function, but too much can kill nerve cells. There are several kinds of receptors that are triggered by glutamate. The ones of most interest in psychiatry are NMDA (N-methyl-d-aspartate) and AMPA (alpha-amino-3-hydroxy-5-methyl-4-isoxazole-propionic acid). It is anticipated that regulating the effect of glutamate will be increasingly important in a wide variety of psychiatric disorders, from Alzheimer's disease to schizophrenia, and that medications that target NMDA and AMPA receptors will be developed over the next few years.

Norepinephrine

As noted, another name for noradrenalin is *norepinephrine*. Receptors for this neurotransmitter are involved in depression and the ability to experience positive feelings. Most antidepressants affect either norepinephrine or serotonin in complicated ways. It used to be believed that antidepressants worked by simply blocking the deactivation of these neurotransmitters, effectively increasing the amount available. This view is an oversimplification: The actual mechanism of action of these medications starts with affecting norepinephrine receptors, which then exert effects throughout the nerve cell. In addition to its effect on depression, norepinephrine is also connected to some pain pathways, and medications that affect this system can help with certain kinds of chronic or neurogenic pain.

Serotonin

Abbreviated 5-HT for 5-hydroxytryptamine, serotonin is a neurotransmitter that is involved in depression, psychosis, and obsessive–compulsive disorder. An increasing number of newer medications target different parts of this very complicated neurotransmitter system. There are now 15 known kinds of serotonin receptors grouped into seven distinct families.

A DISCUSSION ABOUT TIME

Everything, including modern medicine, takes time. Clients often give up on a medication or physicians change doses before the medication has had time to stabilize. Understanding the time a medication needs to take effect is an important part of developing a successful treatment plan. Often, the decision to use one medication rather than another is influenced by how quickly the medication works or how long or short a period of time it stays in the bloodstream. There are four areas to consider when asking how long it will take a medication to work:

1. How long will the medication take to get absorbed from the stomach?
2. How long will it take to build up an effective level in the blood (half-life)?
3. How long will it take to get from the blood into the brain?
4. How long will it take to work once it is in the brain?

Absorption

A medication takes time to enter the bloodstream. An intravenous injection shows up in the blood immediately, whereas a pill taken on a full stomach may take an hour or more. Some medications are absorbed much more rapidly than others. Although the absorption time may influence how long it takes for a medication to work, often other variables have much more impact. How much of the medication is absorbed does matter, however. For example, whereas most medications are absorbed more rapidly on an empty stomach, ziprasidone (Geodon) is much more completely absorbed if there is food in the stomach. On the other hand, quetiapine (Seroquel SR) is only long-acting if taken on an empty stomach; with food, it is still effective, but it is converted to regular quetiapine.

Half-Life

When a person takes the first dose of a new medication, the serum level goes up as the medication is absorbed and then falls as the medication is broken apart (metabolized) or gotten rid of (excreted). If a person takes a second dose of the medication before all of the previous dose has left the bloodstream, the second dose will add to the remaining part of the first dose.

Most medications are eliminated slowly enough that the serum level continues to increase over time, even if the client takes the same dose of medication every day. The ups and downs eventually level off at what is called a "steady-state serum level." If the person then stops taking the medication, the serum level of the medication will fall over time.

Half-life refers to how long it takes for half of the medication to leave the bloodstream. If a medication's half-life is 12 hours, that means that half of the amount taken will be out of the body at the end of 12 hours; half of that amount (75% of the original dose) will be out after 24 hours; and half of that (87.5% of the original dose) will be out after 36 hours. It takes approximately five half-lives for a medication that is taken regularly to reach a steady state. If a medication has a half-life of 24–100 hours (such as flurazepam [Dalmane]), and is taken every night as a sleeping pill, the serum level of the medication will continue to increase every day for 5–20 days before a steady state is reached. If a medication has a 10- to 20-day half-life (such as fluphenazine decanoate) and is given on a regular basis, the serum level of that medication will continue to increase over 50–100 days.

Crossing the Blood–Brain Barrier

Even after a medication is in the blood, it may take some time to cross the "blood–brain barrier" and enter the brain where it can take effect. The brain is surrounded by a set of interlocking cells that form a barrier. These cells are highly modified fat cells. Medications that dissolve in fat cross this barrier much more rapidly than medications that dissolve only in water. Diazepam (Valium), for example, enters the brain rapidly, whereas oxazepam (Serax), a benzodiazepine that is less fat-soluble, takes longer. Large molecules that are not fat soluble may not enter the brain at all, whereas very small molecules, like lithium, may cross almost immediately.

Time to Take Effect

Even after there is an effective serum level and the medication has crossed from the blood to the brain, it takes time for most psychotropic medications to work. We are learning that most of these medications work by influencing the amount of proteins or enzymes that a specific nerve cell makes. It takes up to several weeks for most antidepressants to take effect, whereas side effects often begin almost immediately. If someone taking a medication does not understand this process, he or she may become frustrated by the lack of improvement, feel that the medication is making things worse rather than better, and discontinue it shortly after starting it. If the prescriber does not understand this need for time, there can be confusion about what dose of medication a client really needs. For example, a person who is psychotic is often started on a moderate dose of an antipsychotic medication, but if he or she does not improve within a few days, the dose is often increased. For people who are in the hospital, it is not unusual for the dose of antipsychotic medication to be increased several times during the first week. When the person then begins to respond to this higher dose, it is easy to assume that he or she needs it. Although that may be true, it is just as likely that the person simply needed time to respond and may have responded whether or not the dose was raised.

The opposite occurs when medication is stopped or decreased. The serum level may drop in hours or days, but it may take weeks or even months for the person to feel the full impact of the change. For example, many people with schizophrenia will not immediately become more symptomatic if they stop taking their antipsychotic medication, but they will be at a much higher risk for relapse over the next few weeks or months. In most cases, especially when a medication has been taken for a long time, one should wait weeks to months after decreasing the dose before making the next decrease. A very slow taper decreases the risk of relapse and gives the person the chance to see the effect of one decrease before making the next one.

Drug–Drug Interactions

There is increasing understanding of how one medication can affect other medications. In some cases, one medication can increase the effectiveness of another. For example, lithium sometimes is used to increase the effectiveness of an antidepressant. Similarly, one medication can increase the side effects of another. For example, antihistamines such as diphenhydramine (Benadryl) can increase the tiredness, dry mouth, and constipation caused by tricyclic antidepressants such as amitriptyline (Elavil).

Much recent interest has focused on how one medication can either increase or decrease the serum level of another medication. One medication can influence how rapidly another medication is broken apart and deactivated by the body. For example, carbamazepine (Tegretol) *induces* (increases the activity of) the liver enzyme that metabolizes many other medications, including antipsychotic medications. As a result, if a person already taking an antipsychotic medication starts taking carbamazepine, his or her antipsychotic serum level will decrease. Women taking oral contraceptives and carbamazepine are at greater risk for an unexpected pregnancy, because carbamazepine lowers the hormone level established by the oral contraceptives. Cigarette smoking induces the enzymes responsible for the metabolism of some antipsychotic medications, including clozapine and olanzapine, which in turn decreases the serum level of these medications.

On the other hand, fluoxetine (Prozac) interferes with the metabolism (and therefore raises the serum levels) of many medications, including amitriptyline and diazepam (Valium). If not carefully monitored, a person taking fluoxetine along with a traditional antidepressant such as amitriptyline (Elavil) can rapidly develop a dangerously high serum level of the traditional antidepressant. Fluoxetine has a very long half-life (7–9 days, including its active metabolite), so a significant amount of the medication can stay in a person's body for several weeks. Unless there is a medication-free period of several weeks or the new medication is started at an extremely low dose, the fluoxetine remaining after a switch to a new antidepressant can cause a rapid, potentially dangerous buildup of the new medication. Many of these interactions are not dangerous, but can still lead to uncomfortable side effects. For example, paroxetine (Paxil) can increase the serum level of risperidone (Risperdal). It is not uncommon for a person with schizophrenia to become depressed and be started on an antidepressant. It would be very easy to miss the connection between a person's increased agitation and motor restlessness (akathisia), and the paroxetine that was started a week or two earlier. The agitation could even be considered a symptom of the worsening of the person's depression. In fact, the paroxetine could easily increase the risperidone level enough to be responsible for this new problem.

Some drug–drug interactions are relatively inconsequential, but some may be life threatening. For example, the antihistamine terfenadine (Seldane) was taken off the market because of dangerous interactions. It was very safe when used alone but could cause a life-threatening arrhythmia (irregular heart beat) when taken along with fluoxetine (Prozac) or a number of other antidepressants that interfered with terfenadine's metabolism. Many of the most important drug–drug interactions center around the newer antidepressants (discussed in more detail in Chapter 5). Cigarettes and some foods can also have impact on the metabolism of some medications. For example, smoking cigarettes can induce the enzymes that metabolize clozapine and therefore lower clozapine levels. A person who stops smoking can experience a significant increase in clozapine levels. Grapefruit juice (but not lemon or orange juice) can increase the serum level of a number of different medications, including diazepam (Valium), alprazolam (Xanax), and sertraline (Zoloft).

Drug–drug interactions affect many different medications, and it is one of the areas of psychopharmacology that is most complicated. Information on drug–drug interactions changes rapidly. Pharmacies are an excellent resource for obtaining information on drug interactions. Most pharmacies have constantly updated references and computer programs that can be used to check the interactions between the various medications a person is taking. Most pharmacists are glad to provide information about drug interactions even if the person is not purchasing all of his or her medication from their pharmacies. These tables are provided as examples of some of the most common interactions. They are not intended to be complete. I have noted a Web site in the References at the back of the book that provides updated information about common drug-drug information.

A note about the P450 enzyme system in relation to drug–drug interactions: The CYP450 enzymes, found in the liver, break down and deactivate a large number of substances, including medications and some foods. They are designated by a number followed by a letter followed by another number—for example, 1A2 and 2D6. The first number refers to the gene family, the letter refers to the gene subfamily, and the ending number refers to the specific gene number. The mechanisms of these enzymes are still being worked out, and only a few seem relevant to medications commonly used in psychiatry.

A particular medication can induce (increase the activity of) an enzyme or inhibit (decrease the activity of) an enzyme. A substrate is any medication or any other substance broken apart by a particular enzyme. (Note that Table 2.1 does not cover all possible interactions.)

A Brief Discussion about Money

Those of us who prescribe, administer, and monitor psychotropic medications rarely consider how much they cost. Our clients, however, especially those who pay for their own medications, are painfully aware of the costs. The money spent on the medication may be worth it when measured against the increased suffering and dysfunction that would result if the medication were not available. Still, I think that prescribers need to become more aware of the financial burden a prescription can impose both for the individual patient and for the health care system. In 2000, 6% of the prescriptions written for Wisconsin Medical Assistance recipients were for antipsychotic medications, but these prescriptions cost 15% of the total pharmacy budget for the year. Sometimes less expensive alternatives are just as effective as newer, brand-name medications. Many medications are now available as less expensive generic medications; most of the SSRI antidepressants such as fluoxetine (Prozac) and citalopram (Celexa); two of the atypical antipsychotic medications, clozapine (Clozaril) and risperidone (Risperdal); and most of the benzodiazepines and zolpidem (Ambien) There is still debate about whether generic medications are as good as the brand-name equivalents. When I am prescribed medication by my physician, I use generic medications when they are available. I am comfortable using generic medications myself, and I am also comfortable prescribing generic medications for my patients. Although some people report problems when switched to the generic version of a medication, serious repercussions from the use of generic medications are very rare. The vast majority of people can use generic and brand-name equivalent medications interchangeably, with no real difference except for cost.

Pharmaceutical companies have a natural tendency to try and demonstrate that their newer, more expensive medications are better, more effective, or have fewer side effects than some of these older medications now available as generic. Sometimes these newer medications really are better in some important way, but sometimes the differences are trivial. Unfortunately, it can be very difficult to figure out when the differences are worth the extra cost for the newer medications. Some of the research sponsored by pharmaceutical companies is set up to show a difference when none really exists—for example, by not using a really equivalent dose of two medications being compared, by magnifying differences that are clinically insignificant, or by stressing those results that showed an advantage of the newer medication, but not stressing results that showed the opposite. The bottom line is that the specifics of the research methodology are very important when medications are being compared, but understanding the impact of these specifics is both time-consuming and complicated. Although some of the newer medications are indeed better then those they replace, it is worth keeping an open and somewhat cynical perspective when the overwhelming superiority of a new medication is touted.

TABLE 2.1. *Interactions Between the P450 System and Common Psychotropic Medications*

	QUANTITY	BRAND NAME	GENERIC

Substrates (enzymes listed are needed to metabolize the listed medications)

1A2	2B6	2C19	2D6	3A
clozapine imipramine	bupropion methadone	diazepam amitriptyline haloperidol risperidone codeine venlafaxine paroxetine	amitriptyline clomipramine trazodone sildenafil	buspirone methadone

Inhibitors: these medications inhibit the listed enzymes

1A2	2B6	2C19	2D6	3A
cimetidine fluvoxamine		fluoxetine fluvoxamine omeprazole	bupropion cimetidine duloxetine fluoxetine paroxetine	cimetidine erythromycin grapefruit juice ketoconazole verapamil

Inducers: these medications increase the amount and efficiency of the listed enzymes

1A2	2B6	2C19	2D6	3A
tobacco	phenytoin			carbamazepine St. John's wort

3

Introduction to Antipsychotic Medications

Antipsychotic medications are effective in treating psychotic symptoms associated with schizophrenia, mania, drug intoxication, and medical conditions. They are not equally effective for all symptoms of schizophrenia. They work best in treating the positive symptoms of schizophrenia, but are only marginally effective in treating the negative and cognitive symptoms of this illness. *Antipsychotic medication* is an unfortunate term because it implies that the goal of the medication is to work against the person with psychosis, when the actual goal is to decrease psychotic symptoms. *Antipsychosis medication* is a more accurate description. Despite these misgivings, I use the term *antipsychotic* because it is part of common usage.

Antipsychotic medications are sometimes referred to as "major tranquilizers"—another misleading classification. Although these medications all have calming effects, their major impact is the decrease of hallucinations, delusions, and psychotic thinking. In general, other medications are safer and more effective if sedation is the sole aim. The term *neuroleptic* is also used for this class of medication, especially for first-generation antipsychotics, but it actually refers to a decrease in spontaneous and complex behaviors, which is a side effect rather than a positive effect of these medications. Antipsychotic medications are often divided into first-generation—chlorpromazine (Thorazine), haloperidol (Haldol), fluphenazine (Prolixin)—and second-generation—clozapine (Clozaril), olanzapine (Zyprexa), risperidone (Risperidone). As noted, these second-generation antipsychotics are also referred to as *atypical* antipsychotics because they have less of the motor side effects that are associated with first-generation medications. Over the past decade these second-generation or atypical antipsychotic medications have largely replaced the older medications.

Although this class of medications is labeled *antipsychotic*, it has many other effects in addition to improving psychotic symptoms. The second-generation antipsychotic medications are all effective mood stabilizers even for people who have never experienced psychotic symptoms. They can be used to augment the effectiveness of antidepressants in some people with severe and difficult-to-treat depression. They can be used along with an SSRI in the treatment of severe OCD (obsessive–compulsive disorder). They also sometimes have a role in the treatment of other anxiety disorders as well as the behavioral problems associated with childhood autism. The bottom line is that these medications are very helpful in a variety of conditions beyond schizophrenia.

When they were first introduced, the second-generation antipsychotic medications were heralded as a major breakthrough in the treatment of people with schizophrenia. Clozapine, the first of these new medications, is clearly a true breakthrough and despite all of its potential side effects, for many people it is much more effective than older medications. It is less clear if the other second-generation antipsychotic medications are really as much of a breakthrough as was previously thought. The second-generation antipsychotics have significant advantages over earlier medication in terms of motor side effects, but whether they are really more effective (other than clozapine) is open to question. This determination depends a bit on what we are hoping the medications will do.

How Antipsychotic Medications Work

Dopamine Pathways and Traditional
Antipsychotic Medications

All currently available antipsychotic medications work by blocking dopamine receptors in the brain. Five different dopamine receptors have been discovered: D_1 through D_5. Current medications, both the older first-generation antipsychotics and the newer second-generation medications, all work by blocking the D_2 receptor. There are four major dopamine pathways in the brain, all of which are blocked by traditional antipsychotics. The first pathway starts in the brainstem and goes to the limbic system (mesolimbic pathway). Any chemical that decreases dopamine in the limbic system in the brain decreases psychotic symptoms. Any chemical that increases dopamine in this part of the brain, such as high-dose amphetamines, increases or causes psychotic symptoms. Antipsychotic medications are effective in decreasing psychotic symptoms because they block dopamine receptors in this limbic pathway.

Unfortunately, there are three other major dopamine pathways. The second pathway starts in the brainstem and goes to the surface (cortex) of the frontal lobe of the brain (mesocortical pathway). Dopamine in the frontal cortex stimulates behavior, thought, expression, and motivation. When dopamine in the frontal cortex is blocked, there is decreased motivation, decreased spontaneity, and decreased ability to persist and follow through with things. Blocking dopamine in this area can cause side effects that exaggerate the negative symptoms of schizophrenia.

The third pathway starts in the brainstem and goes to the basal ganglion (nigrostriatal pathway), an area deep in the brain, under the outer layer or cortex. This is the control system for the extrapyramidal motor system. Voluntary muscle movement starts in the surface (motor cortex) of the brain and travels down nerve tracks that look like pyramids when they go through the base of the brain and into the spinal cord—hence the term *pyramidal system* to refer to the nerve tracks for voluntary muscle control. The extrapyramidal motor system (outside the voluntary or pyramidal system) is involved in setting the correct muscle tension so that the person is not stiff but also does not collapse. This is the system involved in making sure that movements are smooth. When dopamine is blocked in this area of the brain, a person can develop EPSEs, extrapyramidal side effects, including tremor, sudden muscle spasms (dystonias), and motor restlessness (akathisia). When dopamine receptors are blocked for a long period of time, they can become "supersensitive" to any remaining dopamine. This supersensitivity is thought to be the cause of TD (tardive dyskinesia), a potentially permanent movement disorder that is a risk with any antipsychotic medication. Although the risk of developing TD is much less with the second-generation antipsychotic medication, the risk is still not zero.

Finally, there is a dopamine pathway that tells the hypothalamus to stop making prolactin, one of the sex-related hormones. When dopamine is blocked in this pathway, the person's prolactin level rised, possibly causing amenorrhea (breast enlargement and expression of milk-like liquid from breasts in both men and women), along with other sexual side effects such as decreased libido.

Joint Serotonin and Dopamine Blockers:
Atypical Antipsychotic Medications

The atypical or newer antipsychotic medications also work by blocking the D_2 receptors in the limbic pathways, but they do this in a way that leaves the dopamine receptors in the other parts of the brain largely unaffected. These atypical antipsychotic medications accomplish this trick of selectively blocking dopamine receptors by using the brain's own self-regulation control system.

In most brain pathways, serotonin tells dopamine-containing nerve cells to stop producing and releasing dopamine. Serotonin acts like a brake on dopamine release. If these serotonin pathways are blocked, this brake is released and the nerve cells release more dopamine. If *both* serotonin and dopamine are blocked at the same time, then more dopamine is released (because blocking serotonin increases dopamine release), but some of the dopamine receptors are also blocked and are therefore less sensitive to this extra dopamine. If the proportions of serotonin and dopamine blockade are exactly right, then the final level of dopamine activity stays largely unchanged.

It turns out that there is no serotonin control system in the mesolimbic pathway, the one responsible for decreasing psychotic symptoms. The serotonin control system is present only in the other three dopamine pathways. This means that if both dopamine and serotonin are blocked, there is dopamine blockade where we want it, but no functional change in dopamine in the other pathways. By blocking both dopamine and serotonin at the same time, these medications act as though they selectively block dopamine in one part of the brain, while not affecting it in the rest of the brain. This effect, of course, depends on a very careful balance of the competing blockades, making this process all more complicated than this simple sketch would suggest. As already mentioned, there are many different serotonin receptors. The one involved in the dopamine control system is $5HT_{2A}$. (The formal chemical name for serotonin is 5-hydroxytryptamine, or 5HT for short.)

Each of the atypical antipsychotic medications has its own unique effect on a variety of receptors in addition to its effects on D_2 and $5HT_{2a}$. These differences in which receptors each medication affects explains both the differences of one medication from one another as well as some of their side effects. For example, medications that block histamine tend to cause drowsiness, and medications that block both histamine and $5HT_{2C}$, such as olanzapine (Zyprexa), tend to cause weight gain. Medications that do not block these receptors avoid these particular side effects. Finally, the different second-generation antipsychotic medications affect the various receptors in somewhat different ways. For example, both clozapine and quetiapine (Seroquel) rapidly attach to, and then detach from, the dopamine receptors, causing an "on–off" state rather than a more consistent blockade. Aripiprazole (Abilify) and some of the newer medications that are expected to become available in the near future are partial agonists, as mentioned previously, that both partially block and partially stimulate the receptors, rather than just blocking them, as do the other antipsychotics. The bottom line is that the various newer antipsychotic medications are very different from one another. With the exception of clozapine, I have seen no data that convince me that any one of the second-generation medications is any more or less effective than any other. That is, for a *group* of people no one of these medications is any more or less effective than another. For an *individual*, however, one medication may work much better than another.

All of the second-generation antipsychotics are designed to block both $5HT_{2A}$ and D_2 receptors, but there is active research on the role of other receptors in schizophrenia, and it is very likely that we will have new drugs targeting glutamate, NMDA, GABA, and muscarinic and nicotinic receptors. Some of these new medications targeting these other receptors may be designed to help improve thinking or memory more then psychotic symptoms. For the moment, all effective antipsychotic medications, first or second generation, block dopamine no matter what else they also do.

OVERVIEW OF SECOND-GENERATION ANTIPSYCHOTIC MEDICATIONS

There are now six newer or second-generation antipsychotic medications, with more on the way. I generally prescribe one of these newer antipsychotic medications over the older ones. I am more cautious about switching medications for someone doing well on a traditional antipsychotic, but over time I have recommended that even people doing well on an older medication may want to try one of the newer ones. There are a few people who seem to do better on the older medications than the newer ones, and for people who do not respond to the newer medications, going back to a first-generation antipsychotic that is a pure D_2 blocker—or if that does not work, using a combination of both a first- and a second-generation antipsychotic—may make sense.

There are now both first- and second-generation antipsychotics available as a long-acting injection. Haloperidol (Haldol) decanoate and fluphenazine (Prolixin) decanoate have been available for many years. Risperidone (Consta) has been available in injectable form since 2004, and paliperidone injection is expected to become available in 2009. The second-generation injectables tend to have fewer motor side effects and are usually better tolerated by the people taking them, but they can cause more weight gain than the older medications. Until recently, all of the second-generation antipsychotics were very expensive, but the availability of generic risperidone makes at least one medication in this class priced similarly to the first-generation medications. Generic olanzapine and quetiapine are both expected to be available in the United States in 2011.

Clozapine was the first of these new-generation antipsychotic medications to be marketed. It was first used in Europe in 1975, but was then withdrawn because of the risk that people taking it could stop making white blood cells. It was approved for use in the U.S. in 1989 with the requirement that white blood cell counts be closely monitored. Risperidone (Risperdal) was released in 1994, olanzapine (Zyprexa) in 1996, quetiapine (Seroquel) in 1997 and ziprasidone (Geodon) in 2001 and paliperidone (Invega) in 2007. Several others are expected to be released in the next few years. All of these second-generation antipsychotic medications block both dopamine D_2 and serotonin $5HT_{2A}$ receptors. Each of these newer antipsychotic medications has its own patterns of dopamine and serotonin blockade, and different patients respond to different medications. Unfortunately, there is no way to predict who will respond best to which medication. For one person, risperidone may work much better than olanzapine, and for another, olanzapine may work much better than risperidone. If someone does not respond well to one antipsychotic medication, it is well worth trying a second and then a third or a forth before giving up and deciding that medications do not work. Since we have no way of knowing which medication is best for a particular individual ahead of time, trying different medications may be the only way to come up with the optimal fit.

Comparing the Effectiveness of Second- and First-Generation Antipsychotics

Clozapine, the "oldest" of the second-generation medications, is clearly more effective than first-generation antipsychotics in people who have not responded to other medication. Clozapine works better in people who have not responded to other medications, and in those who have a partial response but remain very bothered by psychotic symptoms. Clozapine also has much less risk of causing motor side effects than the first-generation antipsychotic medications.

There is an active debate about which of the second-generation medications, other than clozapine, are really more effective in treating psychotic symptoms than are first-generation medications. A large number of studies, mostly funded by pharmaceutical companies, demonstrate that the newer medications are significantly more effective than first-generation antipsychotics. On the other hand, three large government-funded studies— one from England (Cutlass), one sponsored by the National Institute of Mental Health (CATIE), and one conducted in the Veterans Administration—all suggested little or no advantage of the second-generation antipsychotics over appropriate doses of first-generation medications. All of these research studies, both those funded by pharmaceutical companies and those funded by the government, have complicated design problems that make clear interpretation of the findings difficult. A large and complicated research literature reviews this issue, and I will not attempt to summarize it here.

My own view is that the second-generation medications do have an advantage over earlier medications for many people with schizophrenia, but that this difference for medications other than clozapine may be less dramatic than previously thought. If there were really a big advantage of the second-generation medications, it would have shown up more consistently in the research, despite the methodological limitations of the studies mentioned above. On the other hand, the newer medications *seem* more effective to me in the people that I treat. So I am left with a conflict between what studies show and what my experience suggests.

My experience suggests that second-generation medications have subtle advantages that contribute to improved thinking and an enhanced sense of well-being that better supports recovery for those people who have the social support to take advantage of these benefits. If a person with schizophrenia is in a restricted setting with little support for personal growth or change, the possible advantages of the newer medications may have little chance to be manifest. Second-generation antipsychotics also have less potential to cause motor side effects, and therefore there is less need for a person to take side effect medication (which can cause its own problem with memory and thinking). In addition, it appears that the second-generation antipsychotic medications may help more than first-generation medications with cognitive deficits—problems in thinking and memory and abstract reasoning. These cognitive deficits are more strongly correlated with inability to work and to live independently than are positive symptoms such as hallucinations and delusions. My sense is that the second-generation medications can allow for some modest improvement with thinking and memory that becomes more apparent over a duration of 6 months or a year. For some people, these modest improvements in cognition can lead to big improvements in quality of life.

SIDE EFFECTS OF ANTIPSYCHOTIC MEDICATIONS

All of the antipsychotic medications have significant side effects. The side effects of the first-generation antipsychotics are all similar to one another, and are primarily motor side effects. The second-generation antipsychotic medications have side effects that are very different from one another. The biggest concern from the second-generation medication is weight gain and risk of diabetes, but they vary significantly from one another in their tendency to cause these metabolic problems.

First-Generation Medications

The various first-generation antipsychotic medications are fairly similar to one another. They all function by blocking D_2 receptors, and although they have somewhat different side effects from one another, the difference is a matter of degree rather than kind. The first-generation antipsychotic medications can be thought of as "low-potency," "high-potency," and those in between. All of the first-generation antipsychotic medications are equally effective, but they vary in potency. That is, they all do an equally good job, but it takes different amounts of each medication for them to be equally effective. A 100 mg dose of chlorpromazine (Thorazine) is equal in effectiveness to approximately 2 mg of haloperidol (Haldol). The low-potency medications such as chlorpromazine are more sedating and have more anticholinergic side effects (*anticholinergic* refers to a medication that blocks the cholinergic part of the nervous system) such as dry mouth, constipation, and blurred vision, and cause more postural hypotension (drop in blood pressure from sitting down or standing up suddenly), but cause less motor side effects. The high-potency medications such as fluphenazine (Prolixin) and haloperidol (Haldol) are relatively less sedating, cause less weight gain and fewer anticholinergic side effects. They are also somewhat safer than low-potency medications. However, they more commonly cause extrapyramidal (or motor) side effects (EPSEs), such as tremor, stiffness, severe muscle cramps (dystonia), and motor restlessness (akathisia). Some relatively high-potency medications such as perfenazine (Trilifon) and thiothixene (Navane) seem to have most of the advantages of haloperidol, with a somewhat lower risk of causing EPSEs. Medications such as benztropine (Cogentin) can be used to decrease these extrapyramidal side effects. Unfortunately, these medications do not necessarily eliminate all EPSEs, and they have side effects of their own.

Second-Generation Medications

The second-generation medications have very different side effects, both compared to the first-generation medications and compared to each other. Some people seem more willing to take them than the older medications, although research on medication compliance shows less difference between first- and second-generation medication than I would have expected. As a group, the second-generation antipsychotics are much less likely to cause motor side effects, including motor restlessness. These newer medications also seem less likely to cause TD (tardive dyskinesia), although "less likely" does not mean that the risk is zero. They also often leave people feeling less "drugged." People taking atypical antipsychotics are less likely to develop a "dysphoric response" in which they feel "zombie-like." People with a dysphoric reaction may report that they feel terrible but may not be able to describe what the problem is. On the other hand, some of the second-generation medications are much more likely to cause significant weight gain; elevated cholesterol, and predispose people toward diabetes. Olanzapine (Zyprexa) and clozapine (Clozaril, FazaClo) tend to cause the most weight gain, risperidone (Risperdal), quetiapine (Seroquel), and paliperidone (Invega) cause moderate weight gain, and ziprasidone (Geodon) and aripiprazole (Abilify) tend to cause the least. On the other hand, risperidone and paliperidone cause significant prolactin elevation, which can cause sexual side effects, amenorrhea, and perhaps other problems. Ziprasidone and aripiprazole are most likely to cause akathisia (motor restlessness). Not all people experience all side effects, but knowing which medications are most likely to cause which problems can help all team members choose a medication that would be most acceptable to the person taking it.

Bottom Line

The bottom line is that, despite controversy, I continue to prescribe the second-generation medications for most of my own patients and would prefer them if an antipsychotic medication were needed by a family member. I tend to start with medications that have less risk of causing weight gain and less risk of causing diabetes. As previously discussed, for most people the group of second-generation antipsychotic medications have some advantages over the older, first-generation medications, although some of these differences may be less dramatic than previously thought.

INDICATIONS FOR USE

The primary use of the antipsychotic medications is in the treatment of schizophrenia and schizoaffective disorder. As previously mentioned, they also have a role in a number of other conditions, including psychotic and treatment–resistant depression, bipolar disorder, severe anxiety disorders that have not responded to other treatment, and a handful of other disorders. Some of these uses have substantial research demonstrating effectiveness, while other common uses have little to no good research support. The most common uses will be discussed below.

As noted previously, a comprehensive assessment and diagnosis should be conducted before starting any medication. Medications should not be given just because a person is upset or even because he or she is psychotic. Delirium needs to be ruled out first. In addition, medical illness and drug intoxication need to be considered, as these may present as psychosis.

Schizophrenia: Acute Treatment

Antipsychotic medications are not antischizophrenia medications. They treat some of the symptoms of schizophrenia much better than other symptoms. Symptoms of schizophrenia can be divided into positive symptoms (hallucinations and delusions), negative symptoms (apathy, social withdrawal, loss of spontaneity, lack of pleasure in things), and cognitive symptoms (problems with memory, or making decisions). Although positive symptoms are more dramatic and more clearly associated with "being crazy," negative symptoms and cognitive symptoms cause more disability and are more associated with poor quality of life. It is possible to hold a job if you believe that you are God or are hearing voices, but it is very difficult to hold a job if you cannot motivate yourself to work or if you cannot remember what you are supposed to be doing.

Schizophrenia is a chronic, relapsing illness. It can go through periods of improvement followed by relapse, often in ways that are difficult to predict. The long-term course of schizophrenia is highly variable, with some people doing worse over time, and others doing much better than they ever expected. The important point to convey to individuals with schizophrenia as well as the other people in their lives is that treatment is a marathon, not a sprint. The lives of most people with schizophrenia will be much improved if they can find long-term treatment that includes both medication and psychosocial support that will help them deal with the problems caused by their illness. Every treatment decision needs to consider how it will help the person now, what impact it may have over the coming months or years, and how it interacts with the person's values and beliefs.

Initial treatment for schizophrenia usually targets symptoms and helping the person reestablish control over his or her behavior. This might mean helping the person become stable enough to leave the hospital or recover from a crisis. Antipsychotic medications are sometimes used in the hospital in somewhat higher-than-normal doses to help the person get through the crisis period as rapidly as possible. Often the idea is that more is better. The balance between the need for speed and the risk of uncomfortable side effects must always be considered, but for someone in the hospital, erring a bit high is sometimes thought to be better than erring too low. On the other hand, being too aggressive with the dose of medication may cause enough side effects that the person becomes less willing to take the medication after discharge. There is no convincing data that for most people, a very large dose of an antipsychotic medication works any faster or any better than a moderate dose. For most people,

10 mg of risperidone does not work any better than does 6 mg, and 30 mg of olanzapine does not work any better than 20 mg. There may be more sedation and acute calming with the larger dose, but there are also a lot more side effects. There may be some individuals who do need the higher dose, but for most people the issue is time rather than milligrams. If a person with schizophrenia is hospitalized, he or she is often put on a medication, and if not better in 2 or 3 days the dose is raised, and if still not better the dose is raised again. When the person then finally responds, it seems to demonstrate that the higher dose was needed. Actually, we know that all of these medications take some time to work. It is very unclear whether the person really needed the higher dose, or just needed a bit more time. If a person does not respond at all to an antipsychotic medication after 5–7 days, then it may be time to raise the dose or change the medication. It may take a number of weeks or even much longer to see the full effect of the medication.

It is extremely important to decrease side effects as much as possible if we want people to continue their medication. With first-generation medications and some of the second-generation ones, the side effects can be decreased by simply lowering the dose. Research suggests that many people—even those with severe long-term illness—do well with much lower doses of traditional antipsychotic medication than previously thought, especially if they are monitored closely and given additional medication during periods of relapse. Haloperidol at 10 mg/day seems as effective as higher doses for most people with schizophrenia and causes far fewer side effects. At the same time, there is little point in reducing the dose of a medication to the point where it is no longer effective. The goal is not to get to the highest or lowest dose, but to get to the *right* dose. This is the dose that is as effective as possible in targeting the problems that matter most to the client, with as little side effect burden as possible.

The situation is more complicated with the second-generation antipsychotics. With risperidone (Risperdal) less is better; people often do better and have fewer side effects on 4 mg/day of risperidone than on higher doses. With quetiapine (Seroquel), on the other hand, more is often better; it seems to be more effective as the dose is raised above 400 or 600 mg/day, and now it is being used above 1000 mg day with few problems—it appears that the side effects do not get worse with these higher doses. With olanzapine (Zyprexa) more might be more effective, but more also leads to more side effects. Ziprasidone (Geodon) is much more effective at a higher dose and much more effective when taken with food. Some people may experience more motor restless with a higher dose of ziprasidone, but it is much more likely to be effective when used at 160 mg or more. The dose strategy must be individualized for each different medication and for each client.

Schizophrenia: Ongoing Treatment

The vast majority of people with schizophrenia will have a better, stabler life if they continue to take antipsychotic medication on a regular, consistent basis. Unfortunately, about 20–30% of people with schizophrenia do not get much benefit from medication. They remain very ill, and medication does not help. There may also be a small number of people with schizophrenia who will do well even without medication, but there is no good way to predict who will do well and who will not. Unfortunately, most people who feel they will do well without medication turn out to be wrong. Besides the risk that a relapse will disrupt a person's life, there is increasing concern that psychotic relapse is bad for the brain. Medication can cause various side effects and problems, but it can also help the person manage symptoms, maintain function, and may help to protect the brain. To repeat: Most people with schizophrenia will do much better with regular use of antipsychotic medication.

It does seem that some people with schizophrenia, who clearly needed medication when they were younger, can, with middle age and after a number of years of stability, very slowly decrease their dose of medication and in some cases slowly discontinue it entirely. There is, of course, a risk in discontinuing antipsychotic medication and there is no good way to predict who can safely do this. For most people with schizophrenia, stopping antipsychotic medication significantly increases the risk of relapse. The risk can be decreased by making very small medication changes slowly, waiting a month or two or even longer between changes, and following target symptoms that can help both the person and the clinicians to recognize early signs of relapse.

Attempts have also been made to use a targeted medication strategy whereby the person does not stay on medication but restarts medication rapidly, at the first early sign of a relapse. For most people with schizophrenia, however, targeted medication strategies lead to more relapses, more rehospitalizations, and poorer functioning. For the few people who do well when off medication for periods of time and who are willing to resume taking medication when necessary, this strategy may be possible, but generally this approach seems to lead to more life instability and lower overall quality of life.

Most people with schizophrenia do not relapse immediately if they discontinue antipsychotic medication. Research has suggested that a person with schizophrenia who discontinues medication has around a 10% chance of relapsing during the first month. Of those people who do not relapse during the first month off medication, approximately 10% will relapse in the second month, and so on, with around 10% of the remaining people relapsing every month they are off medication. Some people will go many months before relapsing, but this brief period of stability does not mean that medication is no longer needed.

Agitation

Antipsychotic medications can all be used to help calm someone who is very agitated because they have immediate sedative and calming effects separate from their antipsychotic action. It used to be believed that sedation and calming were connected, that you could not have one without the other. Some medications, such as ziprasidone (Geodon), have fairly minimal sedation but are still very useful in helping an agitated person to calm down. Other medications, such as quetiapine (Seroquel), are much more sedating, which may be useful if sleep were a desired goal. There are important differences between the different medications. Ziprasidone is only effective for acute agitation when taken by injection. Roughly 300 mg of ziprasidone in pill form would be needed to equal the impact of a 20 mg injection. Quetiapine is not available as an injection. A 100 or 200 mg pill will help someone calm down, and in some cases that associated sedation may be useful. A larger initial dose increases the risk of dizziness and other side effects. Haloperidol (Haldol) and aripiprazole (Abilify) can be given either by pill or injection. They are both so well absorbed that there is relatively little pharmacological reason to use an injection. A 1.2 cc injection of aripiprazole will have a clinical effect within 30 minutes; it may take 45 minutes to have a comparable effect from a single 30 mg tablet. On the other hand, the tablet will produce a higher blood level the next day than will the injection. One of the main reasons to use an injection of aripiprazole or haloperidol is because the person refuses to take a pill, or because either the patient or the staff want the "magic" that comes from an injection. This can be "good magic," if the person feels that something powerful and helpful is being done right now, or "bad magic" if he or she feels coerced and controlled in a way that may discourage later voluntary medication use.

These medications will help calm someone even for agitation that is not caused by schizophrenia. Agitation caused by terror, delirium, drug withdrawal, hallucinogen intoxication, mania, or psychosis will respond. On the other hand, there are some limitations to the use of these medications. Despite their widespread application, these medications are often less effective in the agitation sometimes seen in people with developmental delays. They may also be less effective in the treatment of behavioral agitation associated with Alzheimer's disease, and in the frail elderly these medications can increase mortality rate. This is not to say that these medications should never be used in people with Alzheimer's or in those with developmental delays, but it is important to carefully balance potential benefits against risk, and then monitor to see if the medication is really helping.

It generally takes 30 minutes or so for even an intramuscular injection to have enough of a serum level to cause a pharmacological effect. If someone is given an injection and calms down immediately, this response has as much to do with the expectations connected *to* the injection as with the medication *in* the injection. Talking to someone who is upset, helping the person to feel safe and to know what is going on, can all work to decrease agitation. Medication can help, often dramatically, but it takes time and it is not the only tool available to help a person regain control.

A first-generation antipsychotic such as haloperidol, a second-generation antipsychotic such as ziprasidone (Geodon), or a sedative antianxiety medication such as lorazepam (Ativan) will all calm a person in the first few hours, but in somewhat different ways. Used in the ER (emergency room) in someone who is not used to taking it, haloperidol will leave the person feeling tired and less reactive to the world—both of which lead to calming. Ziprasidone tends to calm a person down without making him or her sleepy. Giving a very agitated person an injection of ziprasidone helps the person to calm down enough to have a more reasonable conversation about what is causing the problem. Lorazepam will make the person a bit tired and mildly intoxicated. People who are very upset and agitated will also calm down, often very significantly, if someone is willing to just listen and provide support.

Anything that helps calm down a very agitated person will help him or her become more organized and less psychotic. Calming is distinct from the antipsychotic effect of these medications. The true antipsychotic effects take days to be apparent. The decrease in psychosis often seen within a few minutes after taking an antipsychotic medication comes from helping the person to calm down. A psychotic person who becomes more upset appears more psychotic; conversely, if the person is helped to calm down, either by medication or by feeling listened to, he or she will appear less psychotic.

In the past, people with a diagnosis of schizophrenia who became psychotic and agitated were often given repeated doses of 2–5 mg of haloperidol (Haldol) every 15–30 minutes, either as liquid concentrate, pills, or injection, until they calmed down. Current practice is to give one or two doses of medication and then wait. One or two doses usually decreases agitation and psychotic symptoms as fast as higher doses, and leads to fewer side effects. When additional sedation is required, a combination of the antipsychotic medication and an antianxiety medication such as lorazepam (Ativan) is safe, effective, and more comfortable for the patient than administering a high dose of the antipsychotic medication.

The second-generation antipsychotic medications are rapidly replacing the older medications as treatment of choice in calming people who are both agitated and psychotic. There are important differences between the newer medications, and each has its own advantages and disadvantages. In general, it appears that as a group they cause the same kind of calming as the older medications but with less behavioral inhibition. This behavioral inhibition was really a side effect from the older medications and is often uncomfortable for the patient. Although helping someone calm down might be useful in an emergency, when the person is out of control, feeling "wooden" and without spontaneity becomes a problem when the same medication has to be taken for a long period of time. This and other side effects are often so uncomfortable that people given traditional antipsychotics in an emergency may be less willing to take them later. The second-generation antipsychotics appear useful in an emergency, but since they are much less of a "chemical straitjacket," they must be used somewhat differently.

Acute Mania of Bipolar Disorder

All antipsychotic medications can be used to help people who are in a manic state slow down and feel less pressured. First-generation antipsychotics have been used for this purpose for many years. Although they work, they force the person "down" and are often disliked by people with manic symptoms. The second-generation antipsychotic medications seem to be true mood stabilizers, and in general seem to be better tolerated. All of the second-generation antipsychotics are effective in helping the person with manic symptoms regain better control. As noted, they are all different, and each has its own advantages and disadvantages that need to be considered in deciding which to use. Olanzapine and aripiprazole can be started at a full dose right at the beginning. Risperidone, ziprasidone, and quetiapine all require at least a couple of days to reach a full dose. On the other hand, olanzapine is much more likely to cause weight gain—not a big problem during the few days of a hospitalization but a potentially significant problem over time. Aripiprazole is more likely to cause akathisia (motor restlessness), which can be uncomfortable and discourage the person from continuing the medication. All of the antipsychotic medications are often used along with other mood-stabilizing medications such as lithium or valproic acid (Depakote.)

Although second-generation antipsychotics are now being increasingly used as the treatment of choice for acute mania, there is still be a role for the older medications. The traditional approach has been to use first-generation antipsychotics in a moderate to large dose (e.g., haloperidol at 5 mg once or twice a day) to establish rapid behavioral control until lithium or valproic acid (Depakote) has had time to become effective.

When more sedation and behavioral control are needed, a benzodiazepine (clonazepam or lorazepam) can be given along with the antipsychotic medication rather than increasing the dose of the antipsychotic. This combination often allows for behavioral control with fewer side effects.

Ongoing Treatment of Bipolar Disorder

In addition to their use in acute mania, all of these medications are effective, either alone or in combination with another mood stabilizer, in ongoing treatment of bipolar disorder. There is much less data about the use of these medications than there is for the classic mood stabilizers such as lithium or valproic acid, and the older medications are still considered the first-line treatment for ongoing care. On the other hand, for many people antipsychotic medications have significant advantages either in fewer side effects or more effectiveness.

Many people with bipolar disorder continue to have periods of relapse even when taking medication regularly. There are both data and clinical experience that a combination of medications may lead to more effective mood stability than any single medication. Historically the most common combination has been two different mood stabilizers—for example, lithium + valproic acid. Increasingly, there are both data and clinical experience that combining a mood stabilizer with a second-generation antipsychotic medication is both effective and well tolerated.

Bipolar Depression

Bipolar depression is particularly difficult to treat. Whereas mania is more dramatic and possibly pleasurable for the person, most people with bipolar disorder spend much more of their time depressed rather than manic. All of the second-generation antipsychotic medications have data demonstrating that they can increase the effectiveness of antidepressants in the treatment of bipolar depression. Their role as primary treatment for bipolar depression is less clear. Quetiapine has been demonstrated to be effective for treating bipolar depression when used alone. The other second-generation antipsychotic medications have demonstrated that they augment the effectiveness of antidepressants, but there is less convincing data that they are effective when used alone. It seems a bit unclear at this time whether quetiapine really has antidepressant activity different from than the other second-generation antipsychotic medications, or whether there are just better data for quetiapine. My own best guess is that several of the medications in this class have effective antidepressant activity and will almost always be used in combination with lamotrigine or another antidepressant.

What does seem clear is that people who are depressed are much more sensitive to EPSEs (extrapyramidal, or motor, side effects) than are people with schizophrenia. Generally, these medications must be started at a lower dose when treating someone who is depressed, or the side effects will be intolerable. The dose of medication required is also often much less than the dose required for a person with schizophrenia. The dosage varies from medication to medication, but as a general rule when using an antipsychotic medication with someone who is depressed, *less is often better.*

Although use of a single medication is always preferred, when possible, most people with bipolar disorder end up on multiple medications; they simply do not get sufficient mood stability from a single agent. Combining a second-generation antipsychotic medication with a mood stabilizer can be useful in helping the person to achieve a stabler mood, and it can have a beneficial effect on decreasing both the mania and the depression.

Delusional (Psychotic) Depression

People who are psychotic or suffer delusional depression initially respond much better to a combination of antipsychotic and antidepressant medications than to antidepressants alone. Once the client has begun to respond, the antipsychotic medication can be tapered and then discontinued, leaving the antidepressant for maintenance therapy. Except in very rare cases, antipsychotic medications should not be used as maintenance medication for people who have previously had a psychotic depression but who are not currently psychotic. Nonagitated, nondelusional people with depression often feel worse on antipsychotic medications. Too high a dose of an antipsychotic medication can trigger or exacerbate depression.

Dementia and Delirium

Antipsychotic medication may be beneficial in very low doses (olanzapine 2.5 mg before bed or risperidone 0.5–1.5 mg) for agitated people who are demented or delirious. Concern has been raised about this practice, however. These medications do not work consistently, can easily be overused, and increase mortality in this population of people who are often elderly and frail. Furthermore, research studies have failed to demonstrate that these medications really work. All of this has caused the FDA to issue a "black box warning" on the use of antipsychotic medications in people who are psychotic because of dementia. Before starting an antipsychotic medication, the potential risks and benefits need to be considered and discussed with the person's family or guardian, when available. There should be clear target symptoms of what would constitute improvement, and the medication should be stopped if it is not clearly helping. The dose should be kept low, as higher doses can worsen confusion and behavioral problems, especially in elderly people and those with dementia. Medications should be used only after medical causes for agitation have been considered and ruled out, and after behavioral approaches to the agitation have been tried. Most people with dementia who become agitated can be helped to calm down without the need for medication. I believe, despite the FDA warnings, that these medications have a role in the treatment of some people with agitation from dementia and delirium. This role is limited, and the medication should be monitored carefully to make sure that it is really helping.

Drug–Drug Interactions with Antipsychotic Medications

As previously discussed in Chapter 2, medications commonly affect the metabolism of other medications. A medication can increase or decrease the serum level of another medication, often enough to be clinically significant. Not only can psychotropic medications interact with other psychotropic medications, but they can interact with non-psychiatric medications as well.

Cigarette Smoking and Antipsychotics

Cigarette smoking induces (increases the activity of) the enzymes that break down some antipsychotic (and many other) medications, depending on how each medication is broken apart in the liver. Smokers may need a higher dose of clozapine or olanzapine than nonsmokers, but the other antipsychotic medications do not seem to be affected by smoking. It also means that if someone taking clozapine or olanzapine *stops* smoking, his or her medication serum level will increase, and he or she may develop medication side effects. Caffeine can have exactly opposite effects, although usually not as big. Heavy caffeine use can cause at least some increase in serum levels of clozapine and olanzapine, but it has little effect on other antipsychotic medications.

Other Drug–Drug Interactions with Antipsychotic Medications

There are potentially dangerous interactions between some of the antipsychotic medications and many of the medications used in the treatment of HIV. For example, anti-HIV drugs Norvir and Kaletra both inhibit the enzyme that is used to metabolize clozapine, olanzapine, and risperidone. When used together, the antipsychotic medications should be used at a quarter to a half of the normal dose.

Interactions with Street Drugs

Many people taking antipsychotic medications also abuse alcohol or street drugs. Alcohol and other sedating medications can increase the sedative side effects of antipsychotic medications. Many illicit drugs also have anticholinergic effects that can increase the anticholinergic side effects of the prescribed medications. Finally, many people with mental illness are particularly susceptible to the paranoia- or psychosis-promoting effects of many illicit drugs. Despite this increased risk from the illicit drugs themselves, there are few medically dangerous interactions between normally taken doses of alcohol or illicit drugs and normally prescribed levels of antipsychotic medications.

SIDE EFFECTS OF ANTIPSYCHOTIC MEDICATIONS

Some of the most important differences between the various antipsychotic medications are differences in their side effect profiles. Although all antipsychotic medications can cause extrapyramidal (motor) side effects (ESPEs), and all have at least some risk of causing TD (tardive dyskinesia), these risks vary from one medication to another. For some of the medications in this class, the biggest concern is weight gain and metabolic problems rather than ESPEs and TD. Side effects of general concern for antipsychotic medications are discussed in the following material. Specific concerns relevant to specific medications are discussed in more detail in Chapter 4.

Side effects of antipsychotic medications can be divided into four broad categories: (1) metabolic problems, including weight gain and diabetes; (2) extrapyramidal, or muscle-related, side effects; (3) common, non-muscle-related side effects that are uncomfortable but not life threatening; and (4) rare but dangerous problems.

Metabolic Side Effects: Weight Gain and Diabetes

Many second-generation antipsychotic medications are associated with weight gain. As previously discussed in chapter 2, medications commonly affect the metabolism of other medications. A medications can increase or decrease the serum level of another medication, often enough to be clinically significant. Not only can psychotropic medications interact with other psychotropic medications, but they can interact with non-psychiatric medications as well. Not everyone on olanzapine and clozapine gains weight, but it is common. The exact cause of the weight gain is unclear, but it seems related to carbohydrate craving: People on these medications often feel hungry. Weight gain is a problem for people's self-image and general sense of well-being as well as a significant medical problem. Obesity is related to a range of medical problems, including heart disease and diabetes.

Diabetes, a serious medical illness, is associated with blindness, heart disease, kidney problems, and stroke. Diabetes is more common in people with schizophrenia than in the general population; it is also much more common in people who are overweight. Increased weight increases the risk of developing diabetes. Many people with schizophrenia are overweight from a variety of factors, including poor diet, inactivity, and perhaps factors related to the illness of schizophrenia itself. The significant weight gain associated with some of the second-generation antipsychotic medications is certainly a factor in the increased frequency of diabetes observed in people with schizophrenia.

In addition to the diabetes associated with weight gain, there is growing concern that the second-generation antipsychotic medications, especially clozapine and olanzapine, can cause diabetes even in the absence of weight gain. The medications seem to cause direct changes in how the body handles glucose and insulin.

Extrapyramidal Side Effects

Pyramidal cells are nerve cells in the brain that are involved in the control of voluntary muscle movements. *Extrapyramidal* refers to the part of the central nervous system concerned with control and coordination of muscle movements that is not part of the main pyramidal tracts (hence the term *extrapyramidal*). Extrapyramidal side effects (EPSEs) are much less frequent with the second-generation antipsychotic medications than with the older ones, and within the second-generation category there are significant differences in risk. Clozapine and quetiapine are least likely to cause EPSEs, but all of the antipsychotic medications carry some risk of causing these problems. And although the second-generation antipsychotic medications are less likely to cause TD, *less likely* is not the same as *zero*. All antipsychotic medications can cause EPSEs, and all can cause TD. EPSEs can increase discomfort of and frequently prompt people to refuse to take their medications. The effects are dose related, which means that rapidly increasing the dose of a medication increases the risk of EPSEs, and decreasing the dose of a medication is often an effective treatment. EPSEs are usually treatable, and, except for TD, all disappear when the drugs are discontinued. TD has no reliable treatment and may be permanent, even after antipsychotic medications are stopped. There are five common types of EPSE, although in a person who is agitated and psychotic they may be easy to miss. They may be confused with other parts of the person's behavior, and may not appear as clearly as the descriptions below would suggest.

- *Dystonia* symptoms include sudden, often dramatic, spasms of the muscles of the head, neck, lips, and tongue. Tilted head, slurred speech, or eyes deviated up or to one side are also common. Dystonias can be very frightening and at times are dismissed as bizarre behavior rather than recognized as a drug side effect. Dystonias usually occur hours or days after the medication is started or the dose is increased. They are easily treated with anticholinergic drugs such as benztropine (Cogentin; 1–2 mg orally or intramuscularly, or diphenhydramine [Benadryl] 25 mg intramuscularly for rapid relief). Dystonias are very rare with second-generation antipsychotics.

- *Pseudo-parkinsonism* usually consists of muscular rigidity, mask-like face, and stiff walk with loss of normal arm swing and a shuffling gait. These people often have a coarse, 3-second tremor that is worse at rest than with activity. Pseudo-parkinsonism usually begins after two or three weeks of treatment. Parkinson-type muscle rigidity, at least to the extent that it is grossly obvious, is rare with the second-generation antipsychotics.

- *Akathisia* is a persistent, usually very uncomfortable, motor restlessness that is often unrecognized. People feel that they cannot sit still, that they must keep moving even when exhausted. It is characterized by constant pacing, moving of hands or feet, and a feeling of nervousness. People can often distinguish this motor restlessness from anxiety, and they may say something like, "It feels like my motor is running all of the time." Akathisia is one of the reasons that people discontinue their medication, and has been associated with an increased risk of suicide. Akathisia often becomes more severe if the person is already anxious, but it also can become somewhat better if the person relaxes. This side effect is easily confused with anxiety and with an exacerbation of the underlying psychosis.

Although akathisia occurs less frequently with the second-generation than with the first-generation antipsychotics, it is still relatively common. It is dose related, and is more of a risk when a medication is started at a higher dose, or when the dose is increased. Risperidone and aripiprazole are more likely to cause akathisia, whereas quetiapine and clozapine are least likely to cause it.

When clinically possible, the best treatment for akathisia is often just decreasing the dose of the antipsychotic medication. Some people find that caffeine makes it worse, and that decreasing caffeine use can help. Beta-blockers such as propranolol, benzodiazepines such as clonazepam, and anticholinergic medications such as benztropine (Cogentin) can all be useful, but uncomfortable symptoms may persist.

- *Akinesia* is a motor and emotional "woodenness" marked by a loss of spontaneity in facial expression or gesturing, being "slowed up," or shuffling. Subtler but still uncomfortable parts of this syndrome are seen in decreased social spontaneity, diminished conversation, apathy, and disinclination to initiate normal activity. Akinesia is frequently overlooked and can be difficult to distinguish from the psychiatric illness for which the medication is being prescribed. It is partially treatable with anticholinergic medication, but it can also be resistant to treatment and can interfere with the person's quality of life.

- *Tardive dyskinesia* is typically a slow, repetitive movement of fingers, lips, tongue, or other body areas that usually appears after years of medication use and seems to be related to total lifetime dose of medication. Abnormally frequent eye blinking may be an early sign of TD as a writhing motion of the tongue. If the medication is continued, the TD may progress to rhythmic, disfiguring distortion of the mouth or face. Other parts of the body can also become involved. Once it appears as a full-blown syndrome, it can be permanent. It is estimated to affect 20–40% of people chronically using first-generation antipsychotic medications; it appears more frequently in women, older people, and people having a diagnosis other than schizophrenia. It can often be reversed by early recognition and discontinuation of the antipsychotic medication. There are a number of common scales, including the AIMS (Abnormal Involuntary Movement Scale) that allow clinicians to monitor and track early symptoms of TD.

Some people who get very mild TD find that it never worsens, even if they stay on antipsychotic medications. In other people it can progress fairly rapidly over a period of months to become a very disfiguring and incapacitating movement disorder. It is impossible to predict who is at risk for progression to the severe form and who is not. As more people are treated with antipsychotic agents for longer periods of time, TD is likely to become increasingly problematic.

There is a debate currently underway about the risk of TD with the second-generation antipsychotic medications. It is certainly less than with the traditional medications, but it is unclear if the risk is 1% or 10% that of the older medications.

Benztropine (Cogentin) and other anticholinergic drugs can usually control most ESPEs, but they often make TD worse rather than better. As with other EPSEs, symptoms of TD typically disappear with sleep and are made worse by increased anxiety. Similarly, caffeine often makes symptoms worse, although this effect varies from one client to another.

Common, Uncomfortable, but Usually Temporary or Reversible Side Effects

- *Toxic side effects* can affect anyone taking antipsychotic medications. They are usually dose related and sometimes can be controlled by changing doses, taking most of the dose at night, or switching medications. They include drowsiness, feeling "drugged," sluggish, and unmotivated. They are much less of a problem with the second-generation than with the older, first-generation medications. Drug-induced or drug-potentiated depressions also may occur.

- *Psychotoxic effects* include depression, depersonalization, dysphoria, akinesia, confusion, and somatic delusion. Antipsychotic drugs can makes things worse as well as better. These side effects, which are connected to the feeling of being "drugged," all seem to be much less of a problem with the newer, second-generation antipsychotic medications.

- *Anticholinergic side effects.* Medications that block the receptors of the neurotransmitter acetylcholine are called *anticholinergic.* Although most antipsychotic medications have at least some anticholinergic activity, it is not usually a problem with the second-generation antipsychotics, except for clozapine, which has a lot of anticholinergic activity. Most anticholinergic side effects come from the medications used to treat muscle side effects, such as benztropine (Cogentin) or trihexphenidyl (Artane). Some of the antihistamines, such as diphenhydramine (Benadryl), are also very anticholinergic, as are some antidepressant medications such as paroxetine (Paxil) and amitriptyline (Elavil). The most common anticholinergic side effects include dry mouth, blurred vision, and constipation. Anticholinergic medications block sweating and can interfere with temperature regulation, leaving the person much more susceptible to heat stroke. They can make it difficult to loosen the muscles controlling the sphincter of the bladder, causing urinary retention (a problem more frequent in older men). In overdoses anticholinergic medications can cause a delirium that may look as if there is an increase in the person's psychosis. All anticholinergic medications can interfere with memory, especially in older people, or in those for whom memory is already impaired from some other problem.

- *Eye problems.* Blurred vision is a common, reversible side effect from all of these medications, especially the high-dose medications such as chlorpromazine and clozapine. This is an anticholinergic side effect that is made worse by other anticholinergic medications, including medications used for ESPEs, such as benztropine, or by antidepressants such as amitriptyline. The blurred vision goes away when the medication is discontinued.

Lens opacities (cataracts) are a rare side effect, especially of long-term chlorpromazine and possibly quetiapine use. Thioridazine (Mellaril) has been reported to cause deposition of the pigments in the retina, which can lead to blindness. This is rare in people taking less than 800 mg/day for a lengthy period of time.

- *Alpha-adrenergic side effects.* Adrenaline (or epinephrine) works on two different kinds of nerve receptors, called *alpha* and *beta*. Medications that block alpha receptors can cause orthostatic hypotension (sudden drop in blood pressure when a person stands up suddenly), which can trigger a transient dizziness that leads to a fall. Broken bones due to falls in older people are a frequent problem that is worsened by alpha-adrenergic medications. Alpha-adrenergic effects are worse with low-potency drugs such as chlorpromazine (Thorazine) and thioridazine. Among the second-generation medications, they are more of a potential problem with clozapine and risperidone.

- *Prolactin elevation.* Medications that block the D2 receptor cause an increase in prolactin, a sex-related hormone that can cause breast enlargement and secretion of breast liquid in both men and women. Prolactin elevation also interferes with menstrual periods in women, seems related to decreased sex drive, and over long periods of time may possibly be connected to loss of bone calcium, leading to increased risk of osteoporosis. All the traditional antipsychotic medications increase prolactin, as does risperidone (Risperdal) and paliperidone (Invega). Olanzapine (Zyprexa) can cause prolactin elevation when the dose is raised above 20 mg/day. The other second-generation antipsychotics do not commonly cause significant prolactin elevation.

Rare but Serious Side Effects

• *Blood dyscrasia.* Many medications can cause a partial, temporary block in the production of white blood cells and platelets. This is usually of no clinical significance, and within a few days the system is back to normal. Occasionally the white blood count continues to decrease slowly (leukopenia) in a dose-related reaction without other symptoms. This decrease must be monitored closely, and sometimes switching to a different medication is necessary. If this temporary block is relatively complete and the system does not return to normal, the rapid decrease in white cells and/or platelets quickly becomes life threatening. Such a complete block is relatively more common with low-potency, high-dose drugs (chlorpromazine and thioridazine), and it is much more common with clozapine. It is extremely rare with other antipsychotic medications.

    People are at highest risk of a block in making white blood cells (agranulocytosis) in the first 2–4 months after starting a new medication. Symptoms include weakness, high fever, chills, and a sore throat. A physician should be called and a CBC (complete blood count) ordered immediately if someone develops a high fever or chills within weeks of starting a new medication. The outcome depends on how rapidly diagnosis is made. If the client has a blood dyscrasia, all medication must be stopped immediately.

• *Neuroleptic malignant syndrome (NMS)* usually occurs within a few weeks of starting an antipsychotic medication and is marked by a very high temperature and muscle stiffness. People can easily die from hyperthermia (temperature above 105°) if not rapidly and vigorously treated.

    Any client taking an antipsychotic medication who complains of increased temperature and muscular rigidity should be evaluated for NMS. Other early signs include confusion, increased pulse, and increased blood pressure.

• *Fatal heat stroke.* All antipsychotic medications can interfere with a person's normal temperature regulation mechanisms in hot weather. This is a particular problem with clozapine and other medications that have significant anticholinergic activity. During the 1995 heat wave in Wisconsin, eight people taking clozapine died from heat stroke, including several young men who would not normally be considered at risk.

People on antipsychotic medications, especially low-potency medications such as clozapine and chlorpromazine, are much more likely to suffer a potentially fatal heat stroke. People taking these medications should have air conditioners, fans, or a cool place to go if their living accommodations become too hot. They should also drink fluids to avoid becoming dehydrated.

- *Seizures.* All of these medications lower the seizure threshold, although seizures are rare in people taking them. Still, the lowered threshold is something to consider, especially with people who already have difficultly controlling epilepsy. Some of these medications, such as clozapine, are much more likely to cause seizures than other antipsychotic medications, especially when used in higher doses. Seizures are rarely dangerous (unless the person happens to be driving at the time), but they are frightening to both the person and observers.

Antipsychotic Use during Pregnancy

It cannot be proven that any medication is absolutely safe during pregnancy. These drugs do cross the placenta, but there is no evidence that antipsychotic medications increase the risk of birth defects. There is some recent evidence that second-generation antipsychotic medications—in particular, clozapine and olanzapine—may increase birth size (as adjusted for gestational age). This perinatal effect can be a risk factor for later obesity and diabetes. First-generation antipsychotic medications seem to lower mean birth weight. Although all pregnant women should, as a general rule, take as few medications as possible, pregnancy should not be a reason to completely avoid antipsychotic drug use. The stress of psychosis is also potentially damaging to the fetus, and the various risks must be weighed against each other. These drugs will also appear in breast milk. Again, although there is no absolute contraindication, it is probably safer for mothers taking these medications not to breastfeed their babies.

4

Antipsychotic Medications: Medication Profiles

SECOND-GENERATION ANTIPSYCHOTIC MEDICATIONS

Clozapine was the first atypical antipsychotic medication released. Six other atypical or second-generation antipsychotic medications (risperidone, olanzapine, quetiapine, ziprasidone, aripiprazole and paliperidone) are now on the market (see Figure 4.1), and it is expected that several others will become available over the next couple of years. These atypical antipsychotic medications have a mechanism of action different from traditional neuroleptics, as discussed previously. They cause fewer and less severe extrapyramidal (motor, muscle) side effects. They are less likely to cause tardive dyskinesia. It has even been suggested that clozapine might make already existing TD (tardive dyskinesia) better. Finally, and perhaps most importantly, they appear to be more effective than other antipsychotic medications for at least some people, especially in treating the negative and cognitive symptoms that most interfere with people's ability to work and play and lead more normal lives.

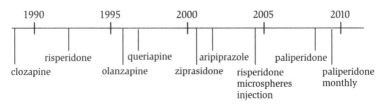

Figure 4.1. Timeline of second-generation antipsychotic medication development.

Clozapine (Clozaril)

Clozapine is the most effective antipsychotic now available. It has too many side effects to use as the first medication tried, but anyone with schizophrenia who continues to have major problems after trying two or three of the other newer antipsychotics should try clozapine before deciding that medications do not work. Clozapine is effective for a significant number of people with schizophrenia who have not responded to other antipsychotic medications. Clozapine is also an extremely effective mood stabilizer and can be used to treat bipolar disorders that have not responded to mood stabilizers. Finally, like the other second-generation antipsychotic medications, clozapine seems to be more effective with the cognitive and negative symptoms of schizophrenia than traditional medications.

Side Effects

Clozapine is the most effective antipsychotic medication now available, but it also has the most side effects. Some are difficult to live with but not necessarily dangerous. The weight gain and other metabolic problems can shorten life span and cause other medical problems, and some of the side effects of clozapine can be life-threatening.

Common, Annoying Side Effects

Clozapine has many side effects, some dangerous and others not dangerous but difficult to tolerate. Sedation and weight gain are the two biggest, most common side effects with clozapine. The sedation often improves over time, but can continue to be a major problem. Drooling, especially at night, is a problem for some people. Clozapine has strong anticholinergic side effects (dry mouth, blurred vision, constipation), and can cause orthostatic blood pressure drops (sudden blood pressure drops when the person stands up suddenly). Other side effects include fever, headache, nausea, drooling, and rapid pulse. While these side effects can be uncomfortable, they are not usually dangerous.

Weight Gain, Metabolic Syndrome, and Diabetes
Weight gain is a very big problem with clozapine. Not everyone on clozapine gains weight, but the average weight gain after a year is more than 20 pounds, which means that some people gain much less than this, but some people gain much more. Weight gains of more than 50 pounds are not uncommon and constitute a major medical problem. Being obese adds to social stigma, interferes with activities, puts increased stress on knees and backs, and causes other orthopedic problems. The biggest problem is that obesity very significantly increases the risk of developing a metabolic syndrome and diabetes.

Metabolic syndrome is a collection of risk factors that indicates that a person is at risk for developing diabetes and other cardiovascular problems, including heart attack and stroke. Metabolic syndrome is strongly associated with obesity. According to the National Cholesterol Education Program Adult Treatment Panel Guidelines (2001), it is defined by:

- Abdominal obesity: waist circumference over 40 inches in men and 35 inches in women
- Increase in serum triglycerides over 150 mg/dl
- A decrease in HDL (good) cholesterol: less than 40 mg/dl in men and 50 mg/dl in women
- Increase in blood sugar of 110 mg/dl or above

Anyone who is obese is at increased risk, especially if the fat distribution is in belly fat. Not all fat is equally dangerous. Fat in the belly is more metabolically active than is fat in a person's thighs or buttocks. This is why waist measurement, more than 35 inches in women and 40 inches in men, is a risk factor. Clozapine (along with other antipsychotic medications) increases cholesterol and serum triglycerides, which also increase the risk for the development of cardiovascular problems, metabolic syndrome, and diabetes.

The most common, medically serious side effect from clozapine is diabetes. People tend to develop adult-onset diabetes as they get older. The risk of developing diabetes dramatically increases for people who are overweight, and as just mentioned, clozapine can cause significant weight gain. Although there is some debate about this next point, it also seems that people taking clozapine (and olanzapine) are at increased risk of developing diabetes even if they do not gain weight. Diabetes is associated with a large number of serious problems, including heart disease, stroke, blindness, and kidney disease. The risk of developing diabetes is a very serious side effect.

There is some very preliminary data that FazaClo, the disintegrating tablet of clozapine that is absorbed in the mouth rather than the stomach, may cause somewhat less weight gain in some people, and may cause less drooling. It is more expensive that generic tablets of clozapine, and these data are still very tentative, but it may be worth trying the disintegrating tablets if these side effects are a problem. There are also some data suggesting that starting metformin, a medication commonly used for diabetes, at the same time that a person starts clozapine, may help to decrease some of the clozapine-associated weight gain. Again the data are still preliminary; metformin is a medication with its own risks and side effects. It seems more effective for preventing the weight gain before it has developed rather than helping the person on clozapine lose weight after the weight has been gained.

Heat Stroke
Clozapine is associated with fatal heat stroke. Some of the fatalities occurred in medically healthy young men who would not typically be thought of as being at high risk. Dehydration and exercise increase the risk. Anyone taking clozapine should be aware of the risk of heat stroke. In very hot weather people taking clozapine should try to find a place to stay that is cool or air-conditioned. They should also take care to drink fluid and avoid excessive exercise.

Seizures
Especially in higher doses, clozapine causes seizures more frequently than the other antipsychotic medications. Although

seizures can be extremely frightening, they are rarely life threatening. An anticonvulsant such as divalproex sodium (Depakote or valproic acid) can be used along with higher doses of clozapine to decrease the risk of seizures, but this added medication increases the potential for weight gain. Clozapine has also been associated with a variety of heart problems and an increased risk of pulmonary embolism. Although these side effects can be extremely serious, fortunately they are very rare.

Agranulocytosis: Loss of White Blood Cells

Approximately 1% of people taking clozapine will develop agranulocytosis (that is, they will stop making white blood cells). If this condition is discovered in time and the medication is stopped, the client can recover without difficulty. If this drop in white blood cells is not discovered, however, the person can die from infections that he or she can no longer fight. There were at least 13 reported deaths from clozapine between 1990 and 1996, even with regular blood testing. Most cases of agranulocytosis occur 6–18 weeks after starting clozapine. Currently, anyone starting clozapine is required to get a regular count of white blood cells to ensure that they are still being made. The purpose of these blood tests is not to determine clozapine level, but to make sure that the person is still has a normal number of white blood cells. "Normal" is considered a total WBC (white blood count) above 3,500, or an ANC (absolute neutrophil count) above 2,000.

In the United States a blood test is required every week for the first 6 months that a person is on clozapine. After 6 months, blood tests are required only every other week, and after a year the screening can decrease to a blood test every 4 weeks. The FDA requires that a person can obtain only enough medication to last until the next required blood test, and cannot receive more medication without first getting another blood test. More frequent monitoring is required for people who have mild decreases in WBC or ANC. Clozapine should be stopped immediately if the WBC drops below 2,000 or the ANC drops below 1,000. Unfortunately, this means that people who do not want to put up with the hassle of weekly tests cannot benefit from the medication. It also means that clozapine can be prescribed only when an organized monitoring system is in place.

Cardiovascular Effects

Clozapine has been associated with myocarditis, an inflammation of the heart muscle. This effect is rare, however, and of most concern during the first 6–8 weeks of starting the medication (although it can occur later). It may present with fever, tiredness, chest discomfort, swelling of the legs, and EKG (electrocardiogram) changes.

Cost

Clozapine is expensive, although the price has dropped now that it is off patent and generic versions have been introduced. A typical dose of generic clozepine (400 mg/day) costs approximately $200 per month (based on charges to Wisconsin Medicaid). The same dose of the brand-name equivalent (clozaril) costs approximately $867 per month. To this must be added the cost of the weekly or biweekly blood tests. There is little reason not to use a less expensive generic when available. Some concerns have been raised that the generic and brand-name products may have slightly different pharmacokinetic properties. This means that as one switches from clozapine manufactured by one company to that produced by another, there *may* be slight differences in serum levels that may be clinically important in some patients. This point is still hotly debated; I have not encountered any problems when clients are switched to generic. Some physicians and some patients have continued to prefer the more expensive brand name because they are uncomfortable risking any change when someone with a serious illness is currently doing well. I think it makes more sense to pay careful attention to any changes in symptoms or ability to function as one switches between clozapine made by different companies, and to adjust the dose up or down as needed. Clozapine blood levels may help make this determination, especially if you knew the blood level both before and after the switch is known. Although some doctors suggest getting these before-and-after blood levels as part of the routine of switching, I generally do not feel this is necessary and most often just follow clinical status.

Specifics of Use

To decrease the risk of seizures and other side effects, clozapine is usually started at 12.5 or 25 mg/day and then increased slowly. In a community setting when we have more time and are concerned that side effects may discourage consistent use, I typically increase the dose by 25 mg every 3 days until a dose of 300–450 mg is reached by the end of 2–3 weeks. In the hospital, where there is more monitoring and more time pressure, it is safe to increase as rapidly as 25 mg a day. The majority of people respond to 300–600 mg/day, with women typically requiring less than men. The maximum dose is 900 mg/day, but seizures are more frequent above 600 mg. It is sometimes suggested that anyone taking clozapine in high doses also take divalproex sodium (Depakote) to decrease the risk of seizures. Divalproex sodium is commonly used in psychiatry as a mood stabilizer (discussed later), but its primary use in medicine is as an anticonvulsant. While adding divalproex to clozapine can decrease the potential for seizures, it significantly increases the risk of weight gain. It is recommended that clozapine be taken twice a day, but in the lower end of the dose range it seems safe and effective to give it once a day if side effects are carefully monitored. There are some data suggesting that clozapine is more effective if the serum level is above 350 ng/ml.

Clozapine may take a long time to reach effectiveness. A person who does not show any improvement at all by 3 or 4 weeks at a full dose is unlikely to get much improvement later. On the other hand, many people who show only a modest improvement initially may have a much more robust response after taking the medication for 6 months or more. If a person does not respond to clozapine, it may be worth trying a combination of clozapine along with a low dose of another antipsychotic. There are also anecdotal reports that some of the side effects of clozapine, especially weight gain and drooling, can be reduced if another second-generation antipsychotic is added and the dose of clozapine is decreased. There is very little research support for combining clozapine with another antipsychotic, but experience suggests that it seems to help at least some people. It is important to stop the second antipsychotic medication after a 4–8 weeks if it has not led to a clear improvement in either symptom reduction, improved function, or decreased side effects.

Drug–Drug Interactions

Clozapine levels are affected by many other medications. Smoking can lower clozapine levels, sometimes a lot. A heavy smoker may require 50% more medication to maintain the same clozapine level as a nonsmoker. This means that a person who normally smokes may require a higher dose of clozapine in the community than in a smoke-free hospital (nicotine patches and inhalers do not effect clozapine level). Caffeine can increase clozapine levels, but this is a much smaller effect than the decrease seen with smoking. Some SSRI-type antidepressants can increase clozapine levels very significantly (e.g., fluvoxamine [Luvox]), but other SSRIs do not affect clozapine levels at all (e.g., citalopram [Celexa]). Divalproex sodium, commonly used as either a mood stabilizer or anticonvulsant, can increase clozapine levels at least a bit. Medications used outside of psychiatry can also affect clozapine levels. For example, the antibiotic erythromycin and the anti-ulcer medication cimetidine can increase clozapine levels to potentially dangerous levels. There may be a slight risk in combining clozapine with a benzodiazepine, especially if the dose is rapidly increased. There have been at least seven reported incidents of people suddenly ceasing to breathe after they were given a benzodiazepine while on clozapine. Given the number of people who have had no problems taking clozapine and a benzodiazepine, the risk of impaired breathing appears extremely low. Confusion, sedation, and increased salivation from the combination have also been reported.

Risperidone (Risperdal)

Risperidone was the second atypical or second-generation antipsychotic medication to be marketed. It is now available as an inexpensive generic medication. It is also available as a long-acting 2-week injection called Risperdal Consta, as a liquid, and as a fast-dissolve tablet.

When used in the recommended dose range of 4–6 mg/day, it has relatively few extrapyramidal side effects (ESPEs), which gives it a major advantage over older medications. Although not as effective as clozapine, it seems to work for some people who have not responded to traditional antipsychotics. It also seems more effective than traditional antipsychotics in decreasing negative and cognitive symptoms. Finally, risperidone may also have some antidepressant activity.

Side Effects

When used below 6 mg/day, risperidone is generally well tolerated with relatively few side effects. The risk of EPSEs increases significantly if a higher dose is used. Weight gain is a problem, although it is significantly less with risperidone than with clozapine or olanzapine. Risperidone commonly causes elevation of prolactin, a hormone that can lead to various sexual side effects, including amenorrhea in women and breast enlargement in both men and women. Orthostatic hypotension (sudden drops in blood pressure when standing quickly) may be a problem, especially in older people, who may fall as a result. The risk of some of the major clozapine side effects, such as agranulocytosis (sudden block in the production of white blood cells) and seizures, seems extremely low.

Specifics of Use

The primary indication for risperidone is for the treatment of schizophrenia and schizoaffective disorder. Like the other sec-

ond-generation antipsychotic medications, it is also useful in
the treatment of bipolar disorder, and can be used in other conditions including treatment-resistant depression, some anxiety
conditions and autism.

Schizophrenia
A full dose of risperidone for most people with schizophrenia is
4–6 mg/day. Two mg/day seems less effective, although it may
be enough for a person very early in his or her illness trajectory.
The frequency of ESPEs, especially akathisia, increases as the
dose is raised above 4 mg/day, and starting someone at the full
dose of 4 mg/day is likely to lead to more motor side effects
than starting at 2 mg and increasing over a few days. Raising
the dose above 6 mg/day increases the risk of akathisia and
other ESPEs considerably, with little apparent increase in effectiveness for most people. Risperidone has a half-life of around
20 hours, which means that most people can take it once a day
without problems.

Mania
Risperidone, along with the other second-generation antipsychotic medications, seems to have true mood-stabilizing properties. Although it can be used alone, most commonly it is used
in combination with other mood-stabilizing medications such
as lithium or divalproex sodium. Risperidone can also be used
for maintenance treatment of bipolar disorder. Using it for this
indication is an important consideration, since it is available in
a long-acting injection that can be taken every 2 weeks.

Depression
Risperidone can be used to augment or enhance the effectiveness
of antidepressant treatment, usually in combination with other
antidepressant medications. It is most often used for agitated or
psychotic depression, but it can also be effective in other depressions that have not responded to other treatment. People who are
depressed tend to be much more sensitive to developing akathisia
and other motor side effects, and the dose used, or at least initi-

ated, should be low. It is may be useful to add 1 mg of risperidone to the regimen of someone who is depressed and not responding well to other medications, and then increasing or decreasing as needed. It is most likely that the dose will need to be raised for a person who is psychotic or very agitated.

Autism
Risperidone is indicated for the agitation that can accompany autism. Typically the medication is started at 0.5 mg/day and adjusted as needed.

Psychosis Associated with Dementia
There is a warning from the FDA that risperidone, along with all other antipsychotic medications, can increase mortality in elderly individuals who have psychosis associated with dementia. There is also concern that using medication to control the agitation sometime seen in this population may not be very effective, and that nonmedication interventions, such as distracting the person or helping him or her stay oriented, may be much more effective. There are times, however, when some kind of medication intervention seems required to allow the person to stay out of the hospital or safe from self-harm or harming others, and these medications continue to be used commonly despite the warnings. Given the risk of using these medications in the elderly, however, it is very important to have clear target symptoms for each medication trial, and then to stop the medication if it is not clearly helping.

In elderly people with agitation associated with dementia, a very small dose of risperidone, usually starting at 0.5 mg/ day and increasing to a maximum of 1.5 mg/day, is often useful. Risperidone and the other second-generation antipsychotic medications have generally replaced haloperidol as the preferred antipsychotic for these patients. Orthostatic hypotension and falls are a potential problem, but the lack of anticholinergic side effects, relatively little sedation, and few EPSEs are all major advantages.

Cost

Risperidone is the first second-generation antipsychotic to be available as an inexpensive generic.

Olanzapine (Zyprexa)

Olanzapine was the third second-generation antipsychotic to be marketed in the United States. It was designed to be more "clozapine-like" than risperidone, and it is well tolerated. It shares some of clozapine's advantages and disadvantages. It works for people who have not responded to other medications, and it seems to be effective on negative and cognitive symptoms as well as positive symptoms.

Olanzapine is available as a tablet, as a fast-acting short-acting injection, and as a fast-disintegrating tablet (Zydis). A long-acting injection may become available. It is expected that an inexpensive generic olanzapine will be available in the United States in 2011.

Side Effects

The biggest problem with olanzapine is its potential to cause weight gain, increase cholesterol, and increase the risk of developing diabetes. It has other side effects including some sedation and some risk for EPSE, but for the most part, other than the weight gain, olanzapine is well tolerated.

Common, Annoying, but Not Medically Dangerous Side Effects
Olanzapine has a low incidence of motor side effects when used below 10 mg/day. Akathisia (motor restlessness) becomes more of a problem when the dose is raised, especially above 20 mg/day. Like risperidone, it has an extremely low incidence of causing a clinically significant decrease in white blood cells. Other possible side effects include drowsiness, dizziness, dry mouth, and orthostatic blood pressure drops. Agitation, nausea, and indigestion are less common but have also been reported. In the commonly used dose range of up to 20 mg/day, olanzapine does not cause the elevation of prolactin seen in risperidone or traditional antipsychotic medi-

cations. If the dose is increased above 30 mg/day, however, prolactin elevation can become an issue. Temporary increases in liver enzymes have been reported but are rarely a significant problem.

Weight Gain, Metabolic Syndrome, and Diabetes
The big problem with olanzapine is weight gain. Average weight gain varies from study to study, but around 22 pounds over 6 months seems to be the mean. In other words, some people gain very little, whereas others may gain much more than 22 pounds. Olanzapine causes about as much weight gain as clozapine, and more than any of the other available antipsychotic medications. The weight gain seems to be caused by carbohydrate craving. Not everyone gains weight, and as with other causes of weight gain, diet control and exercise help. Usually the weight gain starts in the first few weeks after olanzapine is initiated.

Olanzapine carries the same risk of metabolic syndrome and diabetes as does clozapine. Weight gain, by itself, increases the risk of developing diabetes. In addition to the increased risk of diabetes caused by the weight gain, there also seems to be an increased incidence of adult-onset diabetes in people taking olanzapine (and clozapine), even without weight gain. Olanzapine is also associated with an increase in cholesterol and triglycerides, which in turn increase the risk of stroke and heart attack.

The weight gain associated with olanzapine and the other second-generation medications is often very difficult to fight. The initial period of weight gain typically occurs while the person is struggling to overcome or at least stabilize the effects of his or her mental illness, and is frequently accompanied by poverty and restricted activity—which only compound the problem. Informing people about the risk of weight gain, early monitoring of weight, and providing direct suggestions about weight control strategies can sometimes help. It is important to educate the person and support weight control efforts, but not to blame the patient for the weight gain.

There are some data indicating that starting metformin, a

medication commonly used to treat diabetes, can help prevent some of the weight gain associated with olanzapine. This drug seems more effective in decreasing the gain in weight rather than in helping to lose weight already gained, so it must be started before the weight gain becomes significant. There is also some tentative data that Zydis, the fast-disintegration tablet that is absorbed in the mouth, may cause less weight gain than olanzapine tablets that are absorbed in the stomach.

Specifics of Use

The primary indication for olanzapine is for the treatment of schizophrenia and schizoaffective disorder. Like the other second-generation antipsychotic medications, it is also useful in the treatment of bipolar disorder, and can be used in other conditions including treatment-resistant depression, some anxiety conditions and autism.

Schizophrenia

A typical dose of olanzapine for someone with schizophrenia is 10–20 mg/day. In a medically healthy adult, 10 mg can be given as the starting dose, although there will be less initial sedation if 5 mg is used first and then increased after a day or 2. If there is significant agitation, 20 mg can be used safely as an initial dose. EPSEs, especially akathisia, become more common in doses above 20 mg/day. It is safe to increase the dose of olanzapine to 30 or 40 mg, or even higher, but relatively few people will respond to these very high doses if they have not responded to 20 mg.

Mania

Olanzapine, like all of the other second-generation antipsychotic medications, has significant mood-stabilizing properties and can be used as an initial treatment for someone who is manic. An initial dose is typically 10 mg/day but can be as high as 20 mg when necessary to get very rapid control of someone who is otherwise very out of control. It can also be continued for maintenance treatment of mania.

Depression

Like the other medications in this class, olanzapine is helpful in augmenting the effectiveness of antidepressants in people with very agitated or delusional depression, and in people who have not responded to an antidepressant alone. Treatment of depression typically requires a lower dose than that prescribed for mania or schizophrenia.

Quetiapine (Seroquel) and Quetiapine XR (Seroquel XR)

Quetiapine was released in October 1997; quetiapine XR is a longer-acting version of the same medication. It is only longer-acting, however, when taken on an empty stomach; when taken with food, it is converted to the short-acting form in the stomach. Quetiapine XR only comes in larger dose sizes: 200, 300, and 400 mg. Because of the slow absorption and longer half-life, it can be started at 300 mg of the XR once a day and increased over the next few days as needed. A generic version of quetiapine is expected to be available in 2011.

Quetiapine seems both effective and well tolerated. It has the lowest incidence of akathisia and other EPSEs of all of the antipsychotic medications, except clozapine, which suggests that it may have a specific advantage for those people who are very sensitive to these side effects. It causes little prolactin elevation, which suggests that it might have fewer sexual side effects than some of the other antipsychotic medications. It is more sedating than olanzapine but much less sedating than clozapine. Like risperidone, weight gain can be a problem but is generally much less than with either olanzapine or clozapine.

Quetiapine has a primary mechanism of action that seems similar to the other second-generation antipsychotic medications. Each of the medications in this class has its own special properties, however, and quetiapine is no exception. Most of the other antipsychotic medications bind very tightly to serotonin or dopamine receptors; once they bind to the receptor, they tend to stay bound. Quetiapine (and clozapine), in contrast, is only loosely bound. It attaches to the receptor, then detaches, then attaches again. This loose binding may be part of the explanation of why quetiapine is the medication (along with clozapine) that is least likely to cause motor side effects. Quetiapine also blocks some brain receptors that the other currently available antipsychotic medications do not seem to effect as much. One of these is norepinephrine. It is not entirely clear how important this is, but it could explain some of the antidepressant activity of quetiapine.

Side Effects

Sedation is the biggest side effect of quetiapine but is more of a problem when the medication is first started or the dose is increased too rapidly, and tends to be less of a problem over time. Dizziness may also occur in the initiation phase. Quetiapine also causes a slight increase in pulse and a temporary release of enzymes from the liver into the blood. This increase in circulating liver enzymes is reported as an abnormality in some tests of liver function. These effects are seldom problematic. Orthostatic hypotension (temporary drop in blood pressure when standing suddenly) is a problem for some people, as is weight gain. The weight gain with quetiapine is less than that caused by olanzapine but probably a bit more than that caused by risperidone.

Animal testing suggested that quetiapine might be associated with an increased frequency of developing cataracts. It does not seem as though this is really a problem in clinical use, but the FDA recommendation is that people taking quetiapine get baseline and then regular eye exams. I feel that this is more a medical/legal issue than a clinical issue. There is no clinical data from its use with people that the risk of cataracts is significantly more than with many other medications. I do feel that everyone should get a regular eye exam, whether or not they are taking medication.

Specifics of Use

The primary indication for quetiapine is for the treatment of schizophrenia and schizoaffective disorder. Like the other second-generation antipsychotic medications, it is also useful in the treatment of bipolar disorder, especially bipolar depression. It can be used in other conditions including treatment-resistant depression and some anxiety conditions. It is not FDA approved for this purpose, but its sedative side effects allow it to be used to promote sleep, and despite lack of research support it is often used to help people with borderline personality disorder stabilize their mood and anxiety.

Schizophrenia
Quetiapine has a short half-life of 6 hours, which suggests that it should be taken twice a day when possible. The official suggestion is to start at 25 mg twice a day, increasing rapidly every day or 2. This low starting dose minimizes sedation and other side effects. For an otherwise healthy adult, it seems safe to start at a higher dose and increase to an effective dose more rapidly. For someone who is agitated or in significant distress, an initial dose of 100 mg is reasonable, and depending on how the person responds to this initial dose, additional medication can be given later that same day. For a very agitated patient one can start with 100 mg, then give another 100 mg in an hour or 2, up to 300 or 400 mg in the first day. There is more dizziness and sedation when a higher initial dose is used, but the dizziness disappears over a few days. Once on an effective dose of quetiapine, most people can take it all before bedtime, when the sedative side effects can be helpful. At times, it is useful to split the dose, giving most of the dose before bed and a small dose in the morning.

Seroquel XR can be started at a higher dose than regular quetiapine. A usual starting dose for the XR form is 300 mg before bed. It can be taken once a day and is only long acting when taken on an empty stomach.

Quetiapine initially had the reputation for being less effective than the other second-generation antipsychotic medications, but this claim was related to using too low a dose. With quetiapine, more is better; 400 mg/day is a minimal effective dose for treatment of schizophrenia, and it is often more effective in doses of 600 mg/day and above. It seems that the sedation and other side effects do not increase as the dose is raised above 400 mg/day, but the medication seems much more effective in higher doses. The formal FDA maximum dose is 800 mg/day, but it is now commonly used in doses above 1000 mg/day, with few problems and increased effectiveness.

Bipolar Disorder

Like all of the other second-generation antipsychotic medications, quetiapine can be used to decrease the manic side of bipolar disorder. The official recommendation is to start at 50 mg twice a day and increase by 100 mg/day; however, it is safe to start much at a much higher dose. With an acutely agitated or manic person, I often start with an initial dose of 100 mg and then give a second pill 30 minutes or an hour later. Depending on how the person responds, I may give 300–400 mg spread over first day, and then increase the dose further by days 2 and 3. The biggest concern is sedation, which can be an advantage as well as a problem for someone this agitated, and dizziness, which can be a problem.

Bipolar Depression

There are also data that quetiapine is also effective for the depressive side of bipolar disorder. Most people with this disorder spend more time depressed than manic, and bipolar depression is often difficult to treat. The dose of quetiapine used in bipolar depression is typically 300–600—somewhat lower than when the target is mania or schizophrenia. It is most commonly used in combination with lamotrigine, another mood stabilizer, or an antidepressant.

Depression

Quetiapine, like all of the second-generation medications can be useful in augmenting the effectiveness of antidepressant medications in people who are depressed and agitated, psychotic, or not responding well to an antidepressant alone.

Anxiety

There are several studies demonstrating that quetiapine in the lower end of the dose range (25–50 mg), can be used in the treatment of anxiety. It is not addicting or abusable, and is not dangerous in an overdose situation. On the other hand, I am concerned about using a medication in this class too casually. Although it (and the other second-generation antipsychotic medications) is effective and generally safe, concerns about the long-term risks and side effects make it a backup medication for anxiety in special circumstances.

Borderline Personality Disorder

All of the second-generation antipsychotic medications are often used "off label" (without FDA approval) for people with borderline personality disorder. The target of these medication is to help stabilize mood, decrease the disorganizing anxiety, decrease "micro-psychotic" episodes, and decrease hyperreactivity to the environment. There is little research on using any antipsychotic for people with borderline disorder. Case reports and open trials indicate that they are effective, but the double-blind controlled trials have generally not found much of an effect. Clinically, I have found that all of the second-generation antipsychotic medications can sometimes be helpful to this group of consumers.

Quetiapine has the advantage, and the disadvantage, of being very sedating. It can help stabilize sleep, but at the risk of causing more daytime sedation. If sedation and help with sleep are a target, then quetiapine may be worth considering. If sedation would be a negative side effect, another medication in this class might be a better choice.

Ziprasidone (Geodon)

Ziprasidone became available in early 2001. It was the first second-generation antipsychotic that was "weight neutral." That is, although some people may gain or lose a few pounds, most people will have no change in weight from the medication. It came on the market when the weight gain and metabolic problems associated with the other second-generation antipsychotic medications were becoming an increasing concern. Ziprasidone is activating for most people, rather than sedating like the other antipsychotics. Ziprasidone also causes no prolactin elevation, which means that it should have fewer sexual side effects.

It is available as a capsule and as a short-acting injection that is very effective in helping to calm an agitated, psychotic person without putting him or her to sleep.

Specifics of Use

Like the other second-generation antipsychotic medications, ziprasidone is indicated for treatment of schizophrenia and bipolar mania. Although it does not have formal FDA indications for other uses, it also seems effective for the same range of disorders as the other medications in this class, including augmenting the effect of antidepressants in treatment-resistant depression and augmenting treatment for bipolar depression.

Some clinicians have the feeling that ziprasidone is less effective than the other antipsychotic medications. In my clinical experience the main problem with ziprasidone is that it is often started at too low a dose and then maintained at too low a dose. The FDA labeling suggests that in the treatment of schizophrenia, it be started at 20 mg twice a day and increased to a maximum of 80 mg twice a day. Ziprasidone is activating at this low dose and does not begin to have antipsychotic effects in most people until it is at 120 mg a day or above. This means that when used according to its FDA label, it causes significant agitation for days before it gets to a high enough dose to begin to be effective. It is more effective and actually seems to have fewer side effects when started at a higher dose. The current dosing recommendation for people with bipolar disorder is to start 40 mg with food, and increase to 60–80 mg by the second day. I often start an otherwise healthy young adult, with no history of heart problems or frequent fainting, at 60 mg twice a day. Since it often causes agitation, it makes sense to take it at breakfast and dinner, rather than right before bed.

It can be increased a day or 2 later to 80 mg twice a day. Some people will do better if the dose is raised still higher, above the FDA limits, to 240 or 320 mg/day. The official recommendation is that it be used twice a day, but my experience is that after an initial period of stabilization, most people will do just as well if they take it all once a day. IT MUST BE TAKEN WITH FOOD. It is not absorbed when taken on an empty stomach.

Since ziprasidone is activating rather than sedating for most people, the early sedation that we have come to expect from other antipsychotics is usually not present. This activation sometimes leads to the feeling that the medication is not working. At other times, sleep problems or agitation can be a problem. Combining ziprasidone with a benzodiazepine such as lorazepam, especially when starting treatment, can decrease this early agitation and insomnia. On the other hand, the lack of sedation can be a major benefit for someone who is actively involved in a recovery program and may like the energy that can come with the use of this medication.

Risks and Side Effects

Ziprasidone does not cause weight gain or increase the risk of developing diabetes. Its biggest problem in clinical use is that it must be taken with food. It tends to cause agitation when used at too low a dose, and can interfere with sleep if a benzodiazepine or sleeping pill is not used. The biggest concerns are its effects on heart rhythm, although in reality this is rarely a problem in clinical practice.

Effects on Heart Rhythm

Concern has been raised about ziprasidone's effect on the heart; specifically that ziprasidone could (theoretically) cause an irregular heartbeat that could be fatal. This risk seems extremely low, and there have been no reports of such a fatal event either published or reported to the FDA. Ziprasidone does slightly increase the time that it takes for the heart to prepare itself for the next beat. After every heart beat, the heart repolarizes or resets itself. If a new heartbeat starts during this repolarization period, it is possible that one part of the heart muscle will begin to contract before the rest of the muscle is ready, leading to a writhing of the heart instead of an organized contraction. If this starts and the heart cannot reset itself, the person can suddenly—and without warning—drop dead. The time from the beginning of the heartbeat to the end of the repolarization period is called the QT interval. Since it is naturally shorter when the heart beats faster, and longer when the heart beats more slowly, the QT interval is corrected for the heart rate. This corrected measurement is called the QTc interval.

There is a theoretical risk that a fatal arrhythmia could develop at any time, but it is more likely if the QTc interval is longer. With a longer QTc interval it is more likely that the next beat will start before the heart is ready for it. Any medication that increases the QTc increases this risk of sudden death. A large number of commonly used medications increase the QTc interval, such as erythromycin (antibiotic), methadone, and quinine. Ziprasidone also increases the QTc interval and therefore increases the risk of sudden death. This risk is greater if the person has heart damage or is taking other medications that that also increase the QTc interval.

The question is, how big is this risk? The risk is real, but it is extremely small. In the initial research involving 4,500 people the incidence of heart problems was about the same with the other medications, which are considered pretty safe. If there are other reasons for concern, such the patient's age, weight, current heart disease, or being on other medications known to have a strong effect on prolonging QTc interval, then an EKG should be obtained before starting ziprasidone. It might also make sense to obtain an EKG before starting ziprasidone on anyone under 16, since kids tend to be at higher risk for these cardiac conduction problems. With a healthy adult, I feel that the risk of ziprasidone causing an irregular heart rhythm is very low, and that an EKG as unnecessary.

Although there is probably some theoretical but very small risk of sudden death with ziprasidone, the long-term mortality from heart disease is actually less than with most of the other antipsychotic medications. Ziprasidone does not cause weight gain or diabetes, both of which are associated with a very large risk of heart disease and other cardiovascular problems.

Common Side Effects
Although it may cause sedation in some people when first started, ziprasidone's most common initial side effects are agitation and insomnia. These effects are likely to can be a bigger problem for people who are already agitated and having trouble sleeping. People are more comfortable and more likely to stay on ziprasidone if a benzodiazepine (e.g., lorazepam) is used to treat these side effects, especially in the first few days after ziprasidone is started. Nausea is sometimes reported, especially after the medication is first started. So far, ziprasidone seems to have relatively few EPSEs (extrapyramidal or motor side effects), but motor restlessness (akathisia) is not uncommon. This effect tends to be dose related, and may be more of a problem as the dose is increased.

Aripiprazole (Abilify)
Aripiprazole is very well tolerated with relatively few side effects. It can cause some weight gain in some people, but like ziprasidone, it is close to weight neutral for most people. Aripiprazole, like all of the other second-generation antipsychotic medications, blocks both serotonin and dopamine receptors, but it has an additional mode of action that is not shared by any of the other currently available antipsychotic medications: Aripiprazole is a dopamine partial agonist. It both blocks and also partially stimulates dopamine receptors, instead of just blocking these receptors, as other antipsychotic medications do. An *agonist* fires a receptor at 100%; an *antagonist* blocks a receptor 100%. A *partial agonist* fires the receptor at some intermediate rate. In lab research aripiprazole activates D_2 receptors at about 30% of the rate of pure dopamine. Theoretically, this means

that if there is a lot of dopamine in an area, aripiprazole would be expected to decrease dopamine activity. On the other hand, if there is very little natural dopamine in a particular brain area, aripiprazole would be expected to increase firing rate.

Although there is little good research support for any unique properties, my experience suggests that aripiprazole does appear to be different from the other antipsychotic medications. Many people taking the medication like the way it makes them feel. People sometimes report feeling mentally sharper or feeling more alive, appearing "brighter" or more engaged in the world. It seems as though it is particularly effective on negative symptoms. Some of my clients who have refused to stay on other medications are willing to continue on aripiprazole. These subtle effects are probably related to increased dopamine activity in the frontal part of the brain. On the other hand, a small number of people with schizophrenia will become more psychotic when started on aripiprazole. This too is probably related to the ability of the medication to increase dopamine in a person who may be particularly sensitive to this increase.

Specifics of Use

Aripiprazole is available as a tablet, a solution to take orally, a rapidly dissolving tablet, and as a short-acting injection. The primary indication for aripiprazole is for the treatment of schizophrenia and schizoaffective disorder. Like the other second-generation antipsychotic medications, it is also useful in both the acute and maintenance treatment of bipolar disorder, and can be used in other conditions including treatment-resistant depression.

Schizophrenia

I often start an adult on 10 mg/day and increase this to 15 mg/day after a week. If the person seems very sensitive to motor side effects or has had akathisia on another medication, or if this is an initial psychotic episode, I may start at 5 mg and increase more slowly. Most people will do well on 15 mg/day. Aripiprazole has a very long half-life of around 70 hours, which means that taking 30 mg every other day is very much the same as taking 15 mg every day. For someone who tends to miss a lot of medication, increasing the dose can compensate for some gaps in taking it.

Bipolar Disorder

Aripiprazole, like the other second-generation antipsychotic medications, has mood-stabilizing properties. Someone who is very manic and who needs more immediate control can be started at 30 mg/day and then generally decreased to 15 mg/day for maintenance. Because aripiprazole is very well tolerated, some people with bipolar disorder do better on it for maintenance than they do on the more traditional mood stabilizers such as lithium or valproic acid. Aripiprazole can also be combined with lithium or valproic acid for a person who continues to have mood swings on a single medication.

Depression

There is now FDA approval to use aripiprazole to augment the effectiveness of an antidepressant in people with treatment-resistant depression. People with depression seem to be much more sensitive to EPSEs, in general, and akathisia, in particular. When using any antipsychotic medication in a depressed person, the dose should be started low and increased somewhat slowly. This means starting aripiprazole at 2–5 mg/day and slowly increasing to 10 or 15 mg if needed. Although it is not FDA indicated for this purpose, it seems that aripiprazole, like the other medications in this class, can be used for bipolar depression. Like the treatment of unipolar depression, the initial dose must be kept low, 2–5 mg/day, to decrease the risk of akathisia.

Side Effects

Aripiprazole generally causes no increase in cholesterol or triglycerides, no prolactin elevation, minimal weight gain, and is activating rather than sedating. It causes little effect on heart function or conduction. It can occasionally cause nausea, though this effect is more frequent and more severe with younger people and with kids, and is dose related.

The biggest problem with aripiprazole is akathisia. About 10% of people will report at least some motor restlessness when the medication is first started. This effect is dose related and can be avoided by starting at a lower dose; it can be treated by lowering the dose. People who are depressed seem to be more likely to develop akathisia than people with mania or schizophrenia.

Paliperidone (Invega)

Paliperidone (Invega) is a metabolite of risperidone, now marketed as a medication in its own right. The advantages of oral paliperidone over risperidone are unclear for most people. It seems to have about the same potential for weight gain and for prolactin elevation as risperidone. It is similar to risperidone in both its effectiveness and side effects. It has a simpler metabolic pathway than risperidone and has less potential for drug–drug interactions. It is packaged in a very high-tech capsule that slowly releases the medication over the course of a day, which may decrease some of the side effects connected to peak serum levels.

Paliperidone is expected to be available some time in 2009 as a long-acting injection that will only need to be administered every 4 weeks.

Specifics of Use

Paliperidone is FDA indicated only for the treatment of schizophrenia, but it can be expected that to be effective in the same range of disorders as risperidone. It comes in 3, 6, and 9 mg capsules that cannot be cut or damaged without losing the properties of the high-tech delivery system.

Side Effects

The side effects of paliperidone are basically the same as those of risperidone. It may cause a bit less akathisia and motor side effects, but the data supporting this are not altogether convincing.

Iloperidone

Iloperidone is a new antipsychotic medication that is not on the market (and therefore not in Figure 4.1) but is expected to be available in the United States in 2009 or 2010.

As we learn more about how antipsychotic medications work, it becomes possible for the chemists to design new molecules that work in very specific ways. Iloperidone is a designed molecule that has a similar mechanism of action to the other second-generation antipsychotic medications in that it blocks both dopamine and serotonin receptors. Because of its effects on different serotonin receptors, it appears to cause little or no weight gain, little EPSEs, little sedation, and little effect on heart function. It promises to be an effective antipsychotic medication with fewer side effects than currently available medications.

Early studies suggest that it is effective and generally well tolerated. In early, very short-term (4-week) studies submitted to the FDA, slightly fewer people stopped Iloperidone because of side effects than did people taking haloperidol or risperidone. The weight gain on Iloperidone was about the same as that of risperidone. Common treatment-related side effects observed with Iloperidone include dizziness, headache, dry mouth, nausea, and insomnia.

It also appears that Iloperidone will be available in a long-acting injection, probably lasting 4 weeks.

Asenapine

Asenapine is a new second-generation antipsychotic medication that is not yet FDA approved for use in the United States. Preliminary research data suggest that it is effective in both the treatment of schizophrenia and bipolar disorder. It blocks both dopamine and serotonin receptors, as do all of the other second-generation medications. Each of the medications in this class has its own spectrum of other receptors that are blocked, making each medication subtly different. The specific possible advantages of asenapine over already available medications are still being identified. It seems effective in people with schizophrenia and bipolar disease, seems to cause little weight gain, and is well tolerated.

Sertindole

Sertindole was developed in the 1990s, but research was stopped because of safety concerns. Sertindole increases the QTc interval in the heart. As previously explained, if this interval gets too long and the new heartbeat begins before the heart is ready for it, it can result in a fatal arrhythmia where the heart stops effectively pumping blood. Although a number of medications have this effect, to some extent, none of the other psychiatric medications has been found to cause dangerous problems in adults. (There continues to be concern that children may be at more risk.) Sertindole increases this interval more than other psychiatric medication, enough to be of significant concern.

It now appears that sertindole may be effective in people with schizophrenia who have not responded to existing medications. Research is now underway, but if sertindole really is more effective and if the risk can be managed, it may be worth using as a backup medication after other medications have been tried. At this time, sertindole is not available outside of a small number of research sites, but it seems likely to be approved for limited use in selected people.

Table 4.1 summarizes the advantages, disadvantages, and specifics of use of second-generation antipsychotic medications.

TABLE 4.1. *Summary of Second-Generation Antipsychotic Medications*

Drug	Advantages	Disadvantages	
Clozapine (Clozaril)	• Works when other medications do not. • Works better than other medications. • Very little EPSEs.	• Weekly blood tests needed. • Agranulocytosis • Side effects: sedation, drooling, weight gain, diabetes, seizures	• Half-life 12 hrs • Typical dose 300–500 mg/day • Smoking decreases clozapine levels

Drug	Advantages	Disadvantages	
Risperidone (Risperdal)	• Generally well tolerated at < 6mg/day. • Produces only moderate sedation. • Available as inexpensive generic • Available as 2-week injection	• Side effects: Prolactin elevation, some weight gain, EPSEs with higher dose. • Need to increase dose over few days	• Half-life 3–20 hrs • Typical dose 4–6 mg/day
Olanzapine (Zyprexa)	• Is well tolerated. • Can be started at full dose. • Provides rapid control of symptoms. • Produces no prolactin elevation.	• Side effects: more weight gain, diabetes, metabolic syndrome	• Half-life 21–54 hrs • Typical dose 10–20 mg/day • Smoking decreases olanzapine levels
Quetiapine (Seroquel)	• Well tolerated. • Produces very little EPSEs. • Produces no prolactin elevation.	• Dose must be increased over time—400–600 mg/day needed to be effective • Side effects: sedation, some weight gain	• Half-life 6 hrs • Typical dose 300–800 mg/day
Ziprasidone (Geodon)	• Produces no weight gain. • Is not sedating. • Produces no prolactin elevation.	• Side effects: heart conduction abnormalities (theoretical risk), agitation/insomnia	• Half-life 7 hrs • Typical dose 120–240 mg/day • Must be taken with food • Not absorbed on empty stomach

Drug	Advantages	Disadvantages	
Aripiprazole (Abilify)	• Produces little or no weight gain. • Is not sedating. • Is very well tolerated.	• Side effects: motor restlessness (akathisia), risk of agitation	• Half-life 75 hrs • Typical dose 10–20 mg/day
Paliperidone	• Produces fewer drug–drug interactions. • Has simple metabolic pathway. • Available as 4-week injection	• Side effects: EPSEs and akathisia, prolactin elevation, some weight gain	• Half-life 23 hrs • Typical dose 3–15 mg/day
Iloperidone			• Half-life 14 hrs • Typical dose 12–24 mg/day

EPSEs = extrapyramidal side effects.

Table 4.2 summarizes the side effects of second-generation antipsychotic medications.

Table 4.2. Side Effects *of Second-Generation Antipsychotic Medications*

	EPSE	Sedation	Weight Gain	Orthostatic (blood pressure drops)	Anticholinergic
Clozapine	+ /–	+ + + +	+ + + +	+ + + +	+ + + +
Risperidone	+ +	+ +	+	+ +	+
Olanzapine	+	+ + +	+ + + +	+	+ +
Quetiapine	+ /–	+ + + +	+ +	+	+
Ziprasidone	+ +	+	0	+ +	+
Aripiprazole	+ +	+	0	+	+
Paliperidone	+ +	+ +	+	+ +	+

FIRST-GENERATION ANTIPSYCHOTIC MEDICATIONS

Chlorpromazine was the first effective antipsychotic medication. Initially introduced in the United States in 1953, it revolutionized the treatment of people with schizophrenia. Although it still has a role, chlorpromazine is very sedating and often causes people to feel "drugged" or "zombie-like"; it is now rarely used as a primary medication. A succession of other medications was developed; all were similar in that they worked by blocking the D_2 receptor in the brain. Since they all worked in very much the same way, it was unusual for a person to respond to one of these medications and not to another. On the other hand, they had somewhat different side effect profiles, depending on what receptors they blocked in addition to the D_2 receptor. For example, chlorpromazine blocked both acetylcholine and histamine, in addition to dopamine. This mechanism of action caused it to be very sedating and led to dry mouth, constipation, urinary retention, blurred vision, and the "druggy" feeling. Haloperidol is the medication most specific for the D_2 receptor, and as a result, causes much less sedation and weight gain.

The biggest problem with all of the first-generation antipsychotic medications was their tendency to cause motor side effects, often referred to as extrapyramidal side effects or EPSEs. Voluntary control over muscles is carried through nerves that run through what look like pyramids in the spinal column. Involuntary coordination of muscles is controlled by nerves that are outside of these pyramids, or *extrapyramidal*. Dopamine is one of the two main neurotransmitters in the extrapyramidal system, and any medication that blocks it will cause EPSEs. The other neurotransmitter in the extrapyramidal system is acetylcholine, often referred to as cholinergic neurons. In the extrapyramidal system, dopamine and acetylcholine are supposed to be in balance. If a medication blocks dopamine, this system gets out of balance. If both dopamine and acetylcholine are blocked, this system can be brought back closer to balance.

First-generation medications are often divided into "low-potency," "high-potency," and "intermediate-potency" categories. Low-potency antipsychotic medications are just as effective as higher-potency ones, but it takes more milligrams of medication to cause the same amount of D_2 blockade. As a result, the dose is typically in the 100s of milligrams instead of the 5–20 mg range of high-potency medications. That is, 500 mg of chlorpromazine (Thorazine) is about as effective as 10 mg of haloperidol (Haldol). The low-potency medications tend to be much less specific in what they block than do the high-potency medications, which means that they block many other receptors in addition to just the D_2 receptors, including histamine and acetylcholine. Blocking histamine (antihistaminic) causes sedation; blocking acetylcholine causes other side effects including problems with thinking and memory, blurred vision, dry mouth, constipation and urinary retention. High-potency medications that are more selective for blocking solely the D_2 receptors, such as haloperidol, tend to cause many more motor side effects, but since they have virtually no anticholinergic action they are less sedating, cause less dry mouth, memory impairment, weight gain, etc.

There are also somewhat intermediate medications that are not quite as selective as haloperidol and as a result have fewer motor side effects, without as much of the anticholinergic side effects as chlorpromazine; thiothixene (Navane) and perfenazine (Trilafon) are examples of middle-potency first-generation antipsychotic medications.

Low-Potency First-Generation Antipsychotic Medications

Chlorpromazine (Thorazine)

A typical dose range of chlorpromazine for people who are psychotic is 400–1500 mg/day in divided doses. It is commonly said that 400 mg/day is a minimal antipsychotic dose for people with schizophrenia, although there is increasing interest in studying the effectiveness of very low doses. There is little research supporting the use of more than 600–700 mg/day. In the past, injections of chlorpromazine were commonly used to sedate very agitated people, but currently there are safer and more effective alternatives.

Thioridazine (Mellaril)

Thioridazine is now rarely used because it has increased risks of causing a potentially dangerous irregular heartbeat that can be dangerous. It is a well-tolerated, sedating medication, previously given in small doses to people who did not have a psychotic illness. Recently it was shown to cause a substantial increase in the QTc interval (increase in the time that it takes the heart to repolarize and prepare for the next beat). Many medications, including ziprasidone (Geodon), cause this increase in the QTc interval, but thioridazine causes this much more than most other medications still on the market. Although ziprasidone is fairly safe, thioridazine has at least a moderate risk of causing sudden death. As a result, thioridazine is now used only rarely, almost entirely in people who have been on it for years and do not want to switch despite the risk. It is used in the same dose as chlorpromazine, except that it should *never* be used above 800 mg/day and only rarely above 400 mg/day because of its potential to damage the retina, causing permanent blindness.

Because it is sedating, it is often given once a day before bedtime. Some people use it in small doses during the day to calm down. It has historically been used in low dose, 10–50 mg, to calm people who are agitated and developmentally delayed, demented, or personality disordered. In a higher dose, usually around 400 mg/day, it is also effective in some people with schizophrenia. In general, an EKG should be obtained before starting thioridazine, especially in anyone who is older, is on other medications that can effect the heart, or has a known heart disease.

High-Potency First-Generation Antipsychotic Medications

Haloperidol (Haldol)

Haloperidol is the most specific and the most potent of the first-generation antipsychotic medications. It has the most chance of causing motor side effects, and the least chance of causing anticholinergic side effects. The dose range is 1–40 mg/day, although current research suggests that 5–10 mg/day is effective for most people with schizophrenia. Haloperidol is chemically a butyrophenome rather than a phenothiazine. Despite this difference in its chemistry, it seems to work identically to the other phenothiazine medications.

Haloperidol is available as a tablet, in liquid form, and as a short-acting injection for emergency use. It also comes in a long-acting injection called haloperidol decanoate (Haldol Decanoate) that can be given once a month. An inexpensive generic haloperidol is available.

Fluphenazine (Prolixin)

The dose range for fluphenazine is 2–40 mg/day, although recent data suggest that the lower end of the range should be used in most cases. This medication is roughly 50 times as potent as chlorpromazine and is a high-potency, low-dose, "least-sedating" phenothiazine. Along with haloperidol, it the most specific blocker of D_2 receptors and has little effect on other kinds of receptors.

Fluphenazine is available as a tablet, in liquid form, and as a short-acting injection for emergency use. It also comes in a long-acting injection called fluphenazine decanoate (Prolixin Decanoate) that can be given once every two weeks. An inexpensive generic fluphenazine is available.

Intermediate-Potency First-Generation Antipsychotic Medications

Thiothixene (Navane) and Perphenazine (Trilifon)

These two drugs are chemically similar to chlorpromazine but are much less sedating and are generally well tolerated. The typical dose for thiothixene is 5–60 mg/day; for perphenazine, 12–24 mg/day. The biggest concern are the extrapyramidal side effects, all of which are dose related, and tardive dyskinesia, which is a movement disorder than can be permanent, continuing even after the medication is stopped.

Loxapine (Loxitane)

Loxapine is an unusual first-generation antipsychotic medication in that it has less of a tendency to cause motor side effects than most medications in this class, and it seems to exert some action on serotonin in addition to its primary action on dopamine. That is, it seems to have some properties similar to the second-generation antipsychotics. A typical dose is 60–100 mg/day. One of the metabolites of loxapine is amoxapine, an antidepressant, so it can be assumed that loxapine has antidepressant as well as antipsychotic activity. It has a half-life of 4 hours. The official FDA guideline suggests that it should be taken twice a day, but as with most medications, if this is not feasible, once a day seems to work about as well.

Table 4.3 summarizes the side effects of first-generation antipsychotic medications.

TABLE 4.3. *Side Effects of First-Generation Antipsychotic Medications*

	EPSE	Sedation	Weight Gain	Ortho-static Blood Pressure Drops	Anticho-linergic
chlorpromazine (Thorazine)	+ +	+ + +	+ + +	+ + +	+ +
fluphenazine (Prolixin)	+ + +	+	+ +	+	+
haloperidol (Haldol)	+ + +	+	0	+	+
loxapine (Loxitane)	+ + +	+ +	0	+ +	+
perphenazine (Trilifon)	+ + +	+	+	+	+
prochlorperazine (Compazine)	+ + +	+ +	+	+	+
thiothixene (Navane)	+ + +	+	+ +	+	+
trifluoperazine (Stelazine)	+ + +	+	+	+	+

LONG-ACTING INJECTIONS

Long-acting injections of antipsychotic medications are underused in the United States. Historically long-acting injectable antipsychotic medications have been reserved for the most treatment-resistant people, especially those subject to various kinds of court orders that mandate the use of medication. This association between coercion and injectable medication is unfortunate. My experience is that many people with schizophrenia, not just those that are most refractory, do better on injectable medications.

Many people with schizophrenia will do better, have fewer symptoms and have less chance of returning to the hospital if they are consistent in their medication use. The problem is that most people miss doses of medication and have gaps when they go off it for various periods of time. This is as true for people with schizophrenia as it is for most people who take medication for other conditions. Inconsistent medication use is the norm, not the exception. Long-acting injections allow for a more consistent medication delivery with fewer gaps. This increased consistency is enough to increase the real-world effectiveness of the medication for many people. A person with schizophrenia who continues to be symptomatic on oral medication may function better on a long-acting injection.

The use of long-acting injectable medication can also allow the person to focus on areas other than medication. For many people with schizophrenia, the major focus of conversations with family or case manager or prescribers is about whether they are really taking their medication as prescribed. Switching to an injectable medication allows the focus of conversations to switch from medication compliance to other parts of the person's life.

Finally, some people prefer receiving an injection every 2–4 weeks to the hassle of taking a daily pill. The need to take a daily pill can be a constant reminder of illness and loss, and a long-acting injection can allow a person to put this concern out of mind for longer periods of time.

First-Generation Long-Acting Injections

Fluphenazine Decanoate (Prolixin Decanoate) and Haloperidol Decanoate (Haldol Decanoate)

Both fluphenazine and haloperidol are available in the United States in both a short-acting injection appropriate for an emergency situation and a long-acting injectable preparation for ongoing use. It is important not to confuse the two. Both are a somewhat thick, oil-based injection that can be painful for some people. A number of techniques can be used to decrease this pain. The best is to use one needle to suck the medication into the syringe and then switch to a new needle for the injection. The decanoate oil is irritating to body tissues, and the use of a new needle keeps medication on the outside of the needle shaft from causing irritation as it is pushing through skin and muscle in the process of giving the injection.

Dose equivalency between oral medication and long-acting injection is highly variable from client to client. As a rough rule of thumb, l0 mg/day of oral fluphenazine is equivalent to a 12.5 mg (½ cc) injection of fluphenazine decanoate every 2 weeks. Ten mg/day of oral haloperidol is roughly equivalent to a 100 mg injection of haloperidol decanoate every 4 weeks (i.e., 10 times the daily oral dose, given by injection every month). There is some difference between the two medications' pharmacokinetic properties (the way drugs are absorbed and metabolized or, in other words, the speed of onset and how long they remain in the body). With fluphenazine decanoate, the person tends to establish an effective serum level of medication within a day or 2. With haloperidol decanoate, there is a gradual, smoother uptake of medication, and it may take several weeks or more to get an effective serum level.

Because of this slow uptake, it is often useful to start haloperidol decanoate with a higher "loading dose" by giving more medication during the first 2 months and then decreasing to a baseline dose. A person on 10 mg/day of oral haloperidol could be given 200 mg of haloperidol decanoate through several injections during the first 2 months, and then given slowly decreasing amounts until a baseline dose of 100 mg/month is reached. Fluphenazine has the advantage of working faster after a single injection but has the disadvantage of having more side effects a few days after each injection.

Haloperidol decanoate stays in the body longer than fluphenazine decanoate. The half-life of haloperidol decanoate is approximately 21 days, which means that it would take five times that, or more than 100 days, for any dose change to completely equilibrate at a new blood level. Most people do well with a haloperidol decanoate injection once a month. The half-life of fluphenazine decanoate is approximately 14 days, which means that injections are typically given every 2 weeks; it would take 40–60 days for any dose change to equilibrate at a new blood level.

Second-Generation Long-Acting Injections

Risperidone Microspheres (Risperdal Consta)

Risperidone was the first of the second-generation antipsychotic medications to become available in the United States. as a long-acting injection. It combines the advantages of risperidone, which is a very effective and well tolerated, with a modern delivery system that is much less painful than the older oil-based decanoate system. Risperidone is embedded into "microspheres" comprised of a polysaccharide matrix that is very similar to dissolvable sutures. As the material is broken down by natural enzymes, it turns into carbon dioxide and water and the risperidone is released. Because these microspheres are much larger than a normal molecule, the injection requires a special needle with a larger inside bore than most needles. It also requires that the risperidone microspheres be kept refrigerated, and the risperidone microspheres and the liquid dilution must be mixed shortly before use.

The time course of the risperidone release is controlled by

the time course of the dissolution of the microspheres. There is essentially no release for 3½ weeks, then something of a spike of release over the next 3 weeks, and all is completely gone by 8 weeks. Most of the release is between 4 and 6 weeks after the injection. This means that after an initial injection, a person must continue on oral medication for at least 3 ½ weeks. It also means that even after taking injectable risperidone for a very long period of time, 8 weeks after the last injection no risperidone is left. This is different from haloperidol and fluphenazine decanoate, for which a small, decreasing amount of medication may continue to be released for months after the last injection.

Paliperidone (Invega) Palmitate

Paliperidone is expected to be available by the end of 2009 as a long-acting injection that uses a suspension of very small "nano-particles" to deliver an even release of medication over a 4-week period. The size of the particles can be adjusted to make medications that can last even longer, but the initial form is a medication that will last for a month. It is a water-based preparation that does not require refrigeration or mixing, can be given in either the arm or the gluteal muscles, and seems to be a relatively painless injection. The medication can be "front-loaded" to speed the time of onset. An initial dose is typically 150 mg, followed by a second injection, usually 100 mg, approximately 8 days later. Injections are then given monthly, with a typical dose of 75 mg/month and a dose range of 25–150 mg. With this front-loading strategy, there is a clinically effective blood level of medication by 5 days after the first injection.

Olanzapine Long-Acting Injection

Lilly is working on a long-acting injectable form of olanzapine that would be given every 4 weeks.

Table 4.4 summarizes the side effects of injectable antipsychotic medications.

TABLE 4.4. *Side Effects of Injectable Antipsychotic Medications*

Drug	Sedation	Anticholin- ergic	EPSE	Orthostatic Blood Pressure Drop
chlorpromazine (Thorazine)	+ + +	+ +	+ +	+ + +
clozapine (Clozaril)	+ + +	+ + +	+ /0	+ + +
fluphenazine (Prolixin)	+	+	+ + +	+
haloperidol (Haldol)	+	+	+ + +	+
loxapine (Loxitane)	+ +	+	+ + +	+ +
molindone (Moban)	+	+	+ + +	+
olanzapine (Zyprexa)	+ +	+	+ /0	+
perphenazine (Trilifon)	+	+	+ + +	+
prochlorperazine (Compazine)	+ +	+	+ + +	+
risperidone (Risperdal)	+	+	+	+
thioridazine (Mellaril)	+ + +	+ + +	+	+ + +
thiothixene (Navane)	+	+	+ + +	+
trifluoperazine (Stelazine)	+	+	+ + +	+

EPSEs = extrapyramidal side effects;
+ = mild; + + = moderate; + + + = severe; + /0 = minimal.

Table 4.5 compares the side effects of first- and second-generation antipsychotic medications.

TABLE 4.5. *Comparison of First- and Second-Generation Antipsychotic Side Effects*

Side Effect	First-Generation Antipsychotic	Clozapine	Risperidone	Olanzapine	Quetiapine	Ziprasidone
Agitation	+ to + +	0	+/–	+	+	0
Agranulocytosis	rare	+ + +	rare	rare	rare	rare
Anticholinergic	+ to + + +	+ + +	+/–	+ +	+	+
Liver enzyme abnormalities	+	+	0	+	+	+ –
EPSE	+ to + + +	0	+	0	0	+
Dose–related EPSE increase	yes	no	yes	yes	no	yes
Nausea/heartburn	+	0	+/–	+	0	+
Orthostatic hypotension	+ to + + +	+ + +	+ +	+	+ +	+ +
Prolactin increase	+ + +	0	+ + +	+	+/–	0
Sedation	+ + to + + +	+ + +	+	+ +	+ + +	0 to +
Seizures	+	+ + +	+	+	+	+
Tardive dyskinesia	+ + +	rare	+	+	rare	+
Weight gain	+	+ + +	+ +	+ + +	+ +	0

Note. Data abstracted from various sources, including Clinical Handbook of Psychotropic Drugs (17th ed.) by Bezchlibnyk-Butler and Geffries (2007).

+ = mild; + + = moderate; + + + = severe; +/0 = minimal; 0 = none.

Table 4.6 summarizes the side effects of medications used to treat schizophrenia.

TABLE 4.6. *Common Side Effects of Medications Used to Treat Schizophrenia*

Side Effect	Description	May be confused with . . .
Akathisia	• Feeling restless or jittery • Needing to fidget, stand up, or pace around	• Anxiety • Psychotic symptoms • Cocaine intoxication • Alcohol withdrawal
Akinesia	• Feeling slowed down • Losing normal spontaneity • No mental energy ("I feel like a zombie")	• Negative symptoms of schizophrenia • Depression
Anticholinergic side effects (physical)	• Dry mouth • Blurry vision • Trouble urinating • Constipation	• None
Anticholinergic side effects (mental)	• Memory difficulties • Confusion (feeling "spacey") • Visual hallucinations	• Symptoms of schizophrenia • Drug intoxication • Depression
Dystonia	• Sudden muscle spasm; charley-horse (usually happens when antipsychotic medication is started or dose raised; most common with high-potency traditional antipsychotics)	• Strange movements that occur during psychotic episodes in response to stress and may be mistaken for hysterical reactions or malingering

Side Effect	Description	May be confused with . . .
Sexual and menstrual difficulties	• Loss of sexual desire • Loss of erection or ejaculation • Cessation of menses	• Low sex drive can also be due to schizophrenia or depression • Menstrual irregularities often caused by medications and rarely directly caused by schizophrenia
Tardive dyskinesia	• Writhing movements of mouth, tongue, or hands, or any other repetitive movements	• Tremor • Transient movements associated with antipsychotic dose reductions • Spontaneous movements seen in people with schizophrenia even without medication exposure
Tremor	• Shaking of hands or other parts of body	

5

Antidepressant Medications

Antidepressant medications can be very effective in the treatment of depression. However, medication alone is rarely enough. Many people who are depressed are overwhelmed by life stresses. It may be unclear if the depression makes it impossible for the person to effectively cope with these stresses, or if the life stresses are causing the depression, but in most cases, both are true. There is an interaction between a person's biological predisposition to become depressed, and the life stresses that the person is experiencing. While medication is not likely to change a person's life, medication can often help the person to cope with life more effectively. Antidepressant medication is much more likely to be effective if the person taking it understands that the medication may help, but there is likely to be a lot of other work that he or she will need to do as well. The medication is much more likely to be effective if the person taking it sees medication as something that can help summon their energy, focus, or motivation to cope more effectively with real life issues that will not be changed by taking a pill. On the other hand, medication can help with a better night's sleep, more energy, hope, and concentration, and the ability to feel enjoyment. These can all help a person feel less overwhelmed and less hopeless, and allow more effective coping to occur.

There are other effective treatments for depression in addition to medication. Psychotherapy, including cognitive–behavioral therapy (CBT) and interpersonal therapy (IPT), have been subject to controlled research demonstrating that they are effective. Psychotherapy can work to increase the effectiveness of medication and vice versa. There are also a number of excellent self-help books that are based on modern, research-based principles of psychotherapy. In the area of biological treatment, both bright light therapy for seasonal affective disorder and electroconvulsive therapy (ECT) for very severe or delusional depression are effective. Regular exercise has also been demonstrated to be an effective treatment for depression. Although this book focuses on medication, effective treatment of depression requires a much more comprehensive approach to the problem.

Other medications not labeled as antidepressants can be very helpful for people who do not have a complete remission with antidepressants alone. Mood stabilizers such as lithium, thyroid medications such as Cytomel (T3), or a low dose of a second-generation antipsychotic medication can help augment the effectiveness of antidepressant medications. Stimulants such as amphetamines can be effective in treatment-resistant depression, especially in people who are elderly or medically ill. Even a medication that only stabilizes sleep can help someone cope with his or her depression more effectively.

Although this chapter is about medications that are labeled "antidepressants," these same medications can be used to treat a variety of other conditions. For example, the SSRIs (selective serotonin reuptake inhibitors) and the SNRIs (serotonin and norepinephrine reuptake inhibitors) are very effective in the treatment of generalized anxiety, panic, and obsessive–compulsive disorders, bulimia and fibromyalgia. The SNRIs are effective in certain kinds of neuropathic pain (caused by irritation or damage to nerves). Bupropion (Wellbutrin), in combination with a behavioral program, can help people to stop smoking.

CLASSES OF ANTIDEPRESSANTS

Antidepressant medications are divided into five large classes.

1. Antidepressants that work primarily by blocking the reuptake of either serotonin alone—SSRIs such as fluoxetine (Prozac) and citalopram (Celexa)—or by blocking the reuptake of both

serotonin and norepinephrine—SNRIs such as venlafaxine (Effexor) or duloxetine (Cymbalta).

2. Antidepressant that affects serotonin presynaptically (in that part of the cell that controls how much serotonin is released) (mirtazapine [Remeron]).

3. An antidepressant bupropion (Wellbutrin), that works through the dopamine system, but whose exact mechanism is not completely clear.

4. Antidepressants that primarily work to block the reuptake of norepinephrine, but affect a number of other receptors as well—tricyclics such as desipramine (Norpramin) and nortriptyline (Pamelor).

5. Drugs that inhibit the production of monamine oxides—monoamine oxidase inhibitors (MAOIs), such as phenelzine (Nardil), and tranylcypromine (Parnate), and the selegiline patch (Emsam).

   In addition, a number of other medications can increase the effectiveness of antidepressant medications in some clients.

Medications within any one class are more similar to each other than they are different, and although there are some important type differences within a class, these are primarily differences in side effects. As with the antipsychotic medications, some people respond much better to one medication than to another, even if the medications are similar and from the same class. Someone who does not respond to one SSRI may respond well to another SSRI.

At times, antidepressant medications seem to stop working. This "poop out" effect is not uncommon, although the cause is not clear. Raising the dose of the medication or switching to another antidepressant is often effective.

Some people with chronic or recurrent depression do better if they stay on an antidepressant medication indefinitely. The older generation of antidepressants had so many side effects and made people feel so drugged that they stopped them as soon as possible. The newer antidepressants are much easier to tolerate. They still have side effects and risks, but for most people the side effects of the SSRIs and other newer medications are much easier to live with than those of the older tricyclics. People who have had a single depressive episode can often discontinue antidepressant medication after 6–12 months, and although they may be at risk for another period of depression later in their life, they are likely to do well for years without medication. People with a history of multiple episodes of depression, or who have a chronic depression, may do better if they stay on antidepressant medication for a long period of time. This is an individual decision. A large number of people continue on antidepressant medications indefinitely because they feel that their life is better when they take them.

Because the SSRIs have side effects that are easier to tolerate, people tend to take them for less severe depressions. SSRIs are often used for chronic, "low-grade" depressions that cause discomfort but do not interfere with normal function. For these people, the world is not quite as bright as it is for others, roses do not smell as sweet, and things are not as much fun. Is it treatment of an illness or changing a depressive personality if an antidepressant helps one of these people feel happier and enjoy things more? Is this use of medication correcting a problem of biology so that the person can feel enjoyment more normally, or is it enhancing normal function? These same issues are being raised in a growing area of medical treatment, from the use of stimulants to focus attention to growth hormone to help accelerate growth.

THE BASICS

Before starting any antidepressant, obtain a medication history. What medication has the person tried in the past, what has worked, and what has caused significant side effects? While we label the category of medications as "SSRIs" or "SNRIs," and while as a group they have similar side effects and a similar mode of action, they are also very different chemicals. All of these medications are equally effective for a group of people; however, for an individual person one medication may work much better than another. The best antidepressant to start with is often one that worked in the past for either that person or someone in his or her immediate family.

Always obtain a history of the person's past and current medical illness and a list of medications, including herbs and over-the-counter medications, that the person is currently taking. Many medical illnesses can cause depression, make depression worse, or make treatment more difficult. It is also important to take a history of past and current substance use. Alcohol, which is often taken to "self-medicate" depression, can also cause depression and make it more severe. Cannabis can increase apathy, and the withdrawal from cocaine and stimulants can cause prolonged depression.

Also, before starting an antidepressant medication understand what is happening in the person's life. An antidepressant may still be useful even if the depression seems connected to a life catastrophe, but it is important to target what issues the medication can help with, and what issues cannot be fixed by a pill.

Life problems can precipitate a depression so severe that the person can no longer make decisions, eat, concentrate, or sleep, and sinks into a sense of hopeless despair. A medication may help the person feel the energy needed to focus more effectively on what he or she can do to cope with these real-life issues. The medication is not going to "fix it," but it can help the person overcome the depression so that he or she is in a better position to do the fixing that is needed.

Note on terminology: Antidepressant medications work by affecting one or more of the monoamine neurotransmitters in the brain. *Monoamine* refers to a single (*mono*) amine group that is part of the molecule. The primary monoamines involved in the treatment of depression are serotonin, dopamine, and norepinephrine. *Noradrenaline* and *norepinephrine* are different names for the same chemical. The adrenaline/epinephrine system is referred to as the adrenergic system (base root of adrenaline).

CAUTIONARY CONCERNS

Mania and Rapid Cycling

All effective antidepressants can increase mood instability and precipitate mania in people who are susceptible. Antidepressants can also make "rapid cycling" into mania worse. Some people who alternate between being depressed and manic; all antidepressants can increase the frequency and the intensity of these cycles. There is also concern that antidepressants may be less effective for people with bipolar disorder, which makes the treatment of bipolar depression different from the treatment of unipolar (no manic components) depression.

Most people who are bipolar (manic–depressive) spend more time being depressed than they do being manic. The mania may be more dramatic and cause more major life disruption, but the depression is often more difficult to live with.

It can be difficult to determine if someone who is depressed has a unipolar depression (only depression, no mania) or a bipolar depression (a predisposition to become manic, even if the person is now depressed). It is important to always ask about manic or "hypomanic" (less than full-blown mania but still in the mania continuum) episodes in the past. Even without a history of a manic episode, if the person has a family history of bipolar disorder, then he or she is at greater risk of having a manic episode. Medications that are not traditional antidepressants seem to be specifically effective for people with bipolar depression. The mood stabilizer lamotrigine (Lamictal) and second-generation antipsychotic medications such as quetiapine (Seroquel) are both effective for bipolar depression and have less risk of precipitating a manic episode than other antidepressants.

It is very important to consider the risk of causing a manic episode or increasing mood instability whenever someone with a predisposition toward mania takes an antidepressant. If the risk is very high, it often makes sense to start a mood stabilizer such as lithium or valproate along with, or before starting, an antidepressant. In other situations, especially if the risk of mania seems low, going over the risks with the person and family and developing a list of early warning signs for hypomania may be sufficient.

Withdrawal Effects

All of the antidepressants can cause withdrawal symptoms. Although this withdrawal is not medically dangerous, it can cause people to feel more depressed and irritable, to develop flu-like symptoms, and to have trouble sleeping. Some of the medications, such as venlafaxine (Effexor) and paroxetine (Paxil), can cause more difficult withdrawal symptoms, and some such as fluoxetine (Prozac) generally cause much less. Some people are much more susceptible to withdrawal effects, and some less. A slow decrease (taper) rather than abruptly stopping antidepressants can generally keep this withdrawal from coming a significant problem.

INDICATIONS FOR USE OF ANTIDEPRESSANTS

Antidepressants are obviously used to treat depression but they are also effective in treating a number of other conditions, even in people who are not depressed. Most antidepressants are very effective in treating anxiety disorders. They may also help treat bulimia and chronic pain. Buproprion (Wellbutrin) is effective in helping people stop smoking.

1. Depression

It is difficult to predict which depressed person will respond to antidepressant medications and which person will not. Traditionally, it has been believed that people who are more likely to respond to medication may be experiencing weight loss, waking in the early morning, feeling worse in the morning but better as the day goes on, or suffering from depressions that lack a major reactive component (that is, there is no obvious reason why the person is depressed). Unfortunately, there is little data that confirms these beliefs. A pervasive sense of anhedonia (when things the person used to enjoy are no longer fun) and hopelessness are other classic characteristics of depressed people who are thought to respond to antidepressant medications. Other traditional predictions include a family member who is depressed, alcoholic, or has made suicide attempts.

There are a number of different kinds of depression described in the diagnostic manual of the American Psychiatric Association. Major depression is severe and interferes with the person's ability to function. Dysthymia is a persistent, less intense depression that can stay with the person for years. Although major depression is more dramatic, dysthymia can also cause people to feel miserable, interfere with their ability to feel pleasure, and lead to major problems in relationships. Both are treatable. In most cases treatment involves psychotherapy with either an interpersonal or cognitive–behavioral approach, combined with medication. It often makes sense for someone with dysthymia to start with psychotherapy, but if the depression continues antidepressant medication should be considered.

Antidepressant medications seem ineffective in people going through a typical grief reaction or in those with a depression that seems primarily reactive to life events, although if the person gets "stuck" in grieving or has a significant history of recurrent depression in the past, an antidepressant may be indicated.

Most people with a depression do well with just one antidepressant and do not need a combination of different medications. The goal, however, is not just to decrease the depression, but also to get the person completely over the depression. At times, combinations of medication are needed to accomplish this more comprehensive goal. For example, people who are agitated or have a major sleep problem may respond faster if given an antianxiety medication, such as diazepam (Valium) or lorazepam (Ativan), for a few days at the beginning of treatment, in addition to an antidepressant. Some people with a very agitated depression, especially if they have psychotic symptoms, initially respond better to a combination of antipsychotic antidepressant and medication. People with a delusional depression initially respond much better to antipsychotic and antidepressant combinations than to antidepressants alone. Antidepressant medications can be used safely with antipsychotics, common sleeping pills, or electroconvulsive therapy (ECT), and they are useful in combination with lithium or other mood stabilizers in people who are in the depressed phase of a manic–depressive (bipolar) illness.

2. Anxiety Disorders

These medications are called "antidepressants" because they were first used to treat depression. They are, however, effective for a number of other conditions, and they just as easily could have been called "anti-panic" or antianxiety medications. Most antidepressants are useful for anxiety disorders, whether or not the person is depressed.

We used to just talk about anxiety as though it were a single disorder. It is now clear that there are a number of different anxiety disorders, each with its own biology and each responding somewhat differently to treatment. All of them respond, at least to some extent, to antidepressants, but not all of them respond to the traditional Valium-type antianxiety medications.

The current diagnostic system lists five different anxiety disorders.

- Panic disorder
- Obsessive–compulsive disorder (OCD)
- Generalized anxiety disorder (GAD)
- Social phobia
- Posttraumatic stress disorder (PTSD)

- *Panic disorder.* This disorder is characterized by brief periods of extremely intense anxiety. People may feel as if they are dying or having a heart attack. Panic attacks often occur when the person is relaxed, without any apparent stressors. Typically, people with repeating panic attacks start developing fear of being in places where they may be trapped. As a result they start avoiding crowded places such as shopping centers, or open areas where they cannot return home rapidly. This fear of going out is called *agoraphobia* (Greek for, fear of the marketplace). Panic can be so severe and frequent as to cause major problems in people's lives, and it can be so upsetting and debilitating that it can make some people suicidal. Almost all of the antidepressants (except bupropion [Wellbutrin]) are effective anti-panic treatment. Because they are less addicting and less sedating than the benzodiazepines, antidepressants have become "first-line" medications for panic.

- *Obsessive–compulsive disorder (OCD).* Strongly serotonergic medications, including all of the SSRIs and clomipramine (Anafranil), are helpful, when used in combination with behavioral therapy, for many people who have this often disabling disorder. OCD sometimes requires a higher dose of medication than does depression. For example, 20 mg/day of fluoxetine (Prozac) is generally an effective dose for most people with depression and most people with OCD. Some people with OCD, however, may require 60–80 mg/day. All of the SSRI medications seem equally effective in OCD, although there is less research for some than others. Clomipramine (Anafranil) sometimes works for some people with OCD who do not respond to the SSRIs. I do not use it as my first medication of choice because it has many more side effects than the SSRIs. Clomipramine is sedating, causes weight gain, dry mouth, and constipation, and is more dangerous when taken as an overdose. However, it sometimes helps with OCD when other medications are ineffective. Typically, clomipramine is started at 25 mg/day and then increased to 150 mg/day. A typical dose range for OCD is 150–250 mg/day.

- *Generalized anxiety disorder (GAD).* A number of research studies (and clinical experience) suggest that most antidepressants are useful for GAD. Unlike a benzodiazepine that starts working right away, most people need to take an antidepressant regularly for days to weeks before it begins to be effective. It has less of an initial "kick" than a benzodiazepine, so people may not feel that it is as effective. Benzodiazepines are safe and effective when prescribed and taken appropriately, but the antidepressants are not addicting, and, for the most part, they are less sedating. They may also cause fewer cognitive problems, such as the memory problems that some people report with benzodiazepines.

- *Social phobias.* People with social phobia can become so embarrassed by how other people may judge them that they become virtual recluses. This is a common condition and can interfere with all areas of a person's life. A number of different medications, including most of the antidepressants, can decrease the intensity of the fear.

- *Posttraumatic stress disorder (PTSD).* Antidepressants are commonly used to decrease the depression commonly associated with PTSD and are often combined with other medications to treat the various symptoms of heightened startle response, intrusive nightmares, and overarousal that are common parts of this disorder.

Bulimia

Most of the antidepressants (including all of the tricyclics and SSRIs) can be helpful in the treatment of people with bulimia, whether they are depressed or not. These medications can decrease the frequency and severity of the binging and help people with bulimia to establish more control over their own eating.

Neuropathic Pain

Diabetic neuropathy and other kinds of neuropathic pain (pain caused by damage to nerves), different kinds of pain have different underlying physiological mechanisms. The pain associated with nerve damage seems to involve norepinephrine, and the SNRIs, which affect both serotonin and norepinephrine, can help with this pain even in people who are not depressed. The older tricycle antidepressants such as amitriptyline (Elavil) have been used for pain and headaches for many years. Duloxetine (Cymbalta) has good research supporting its use in diabetic-induced pain and has an FDA indication for this use. Venlafaxine, another SNRI, also seems effective for neuropathic pain, although it does not have an FDA indication for this use and less research on it has been conducted.

Smoking Cessation

Bupropion, used in combination with a nicotine patch and a smoking cessation program, seems effective in helping motivated people quit smoking. This effect is specific to bupropion; other antidepressants do not appear to be effective in decreasing smoking. Bupropion should be started 7–10 days before the designated "stop smoking" day, and the nicotine patch should be started when the smoking is stopped. Generally, a normal antidepressant dose is used. Bupropion can be started at 100 mg twice a day for 3 days and then increased to 150 mg twice a day. Bupropion is marketed under the name Wellbutrin when used as an antidepressant and as Zyban when used as part of a smoking cessation program. They are exactly the same medication.

Fibromyalgia

Fibromyalgia is a persistent condition characterized by widespread muscle pain and tenderness to even light touch. Sleep disturbance, problems with concentration and memory, and fatigue are all common. SSRIs and the SNRIs are effective for some people who have fibromyalgia, decreasing the pain and helping to stabilize sleep, even in people who are not depressed. Antidepressants are also useful for a variety of other conditions. For example, they can be used to treat a variety of what are called "stage-four sleep disorders," which include night terrors and enuresis in children.

TYPES OF ANTIDEPRESSANTS

There are five major types of antidepressants, based on their basic mechanism of action. The most common antidepressants now in use in the United States are the SSRIs and SNRIs that selectively block the reuptake back into the nerve cell, of either serotonin or norepinephrine, or both. An NRI (norepinephrine reuptake inhibitor) is available in Europe. The second type of antidepressant works by increasing the amount of serotonin and norepinephrine released by affecting the releasing, or presynaptic, neuron. The third antidepressant is bupropion, which is in its own class, and increases dopamine, another neurotransmitter involved in depression. The fourth type is comprised of tricyclic antidepressants, so called because of their three–ring chemical structure. They also work by blocking the reuptake of serotonin and norepinephrine, similar to the SSRIs and SNRIs, but they are much less selective, and thus tend to have more side effects. The last type of antidepressant is the MAO inhibitor. This medication blocks monoamine oxidase, one of the major enzymes which breaks apart serotonin, norepinephrine, and dopamine. By inhibiting this enzyme, these neurotransmitters stay in the synapse slightly longer, and thus have more time to have an effect.

Medications That Selectively Affect Serotonin and/or Norepinephrine Systems

Almost all of the currently available antidepressants, with the exception of bupropion (Wellbutrin) work by influencing either norepinephrine or serotonin or both. The first-generation antidepressants, the tricyclics and MAOIs, worked through these same systems but they also affected many other systems throughout the brain and the body, causing many side effects. The SSRI and SNRI antidepressants are much more selective, acting more precisely on the parts of the neurotransmitters that seem related to depression. This means that they are far safer and cause fewer side effects than the older medications. However, although the newer medications may be more effective in treating anxiety disorders than the older ones, they do not appear to be any more effective in treating depression—but they are safer and easier to tolerate.

Selective Serotonin Reuptake Inhibitors (SSRIs)

The first of the new generation of antidepressants—Prozac (fluoxetine)—selectively blocks the reuptake of serotonin and was widely publicized as something of a "miracle drug." It was even featured on the cover of *Newsweek*. Concern has been raised that these medications may increase "suicidal behavior," especially in children and people under 25. The data addressing these concerns are complicated. There is some research indicating that younger people put on an antidepressant are more likely to talk about suicide and perhaps make suicide attempts. There are no data that they are more likely to actually kill themselves, and some data suggest that the SSRIs decrease the risk of completed suicide. The reality is that these new medications are not miracle drugs. For typical depression they are no more effective than the older tricyclic antidepressants. Their major advantage is that they are much safer and are generally better tolerated than the older medications.

How SSRIs Work

A nerve cell communicates with an adjacent cell by releasing a chemical called a neurotransmitter, which activates receptors on that nearby cell. After this release, the neurotransmitter must be disposed of or deactivated before the cell receptors can become active again. There are two primary ways that this disposal/deactivation occurs. One is to break the neurotransmitter molecule into smaller, inactive pieces. The second is to literally suck the neurotransmitter back into the cell that just released it, clearing from the space between the cells, so that it can be repackaged and used again. The SSRIs block this reuptake process, leaving a longer period of time for the serotonin to act on the receiving cell.

These new antidepressants are much more selective in blocking the targeted neurotransmitter than are older tricyclic antidepressants. Although these medications do not appear to be any more effective overall than the older medications, their selectivity decreases their side effects. The serotonergic antidepressants may be particularly useful for people with an anxiety disorder, especially those with an OCD.

The SSRIs are more similar than they are different. For all practical purposes, if one of these medications generally is effective for a particular problem, all of the other medications in this same class will also work for the same problem. For reasons that are not exactly clear, however, a person may respond to one of the medications in this group much better than to another, so it is sometimes worth trying another one if the first does not work. Although the side effects are all somewhat similar, there are some differences in the frequency of different side effects in different medications in this class.

Specifics of Use
- *Fluoxetine (Prozac)* is typically prescribed at 20 mg/day, although older people may not tolerate this high a dose, and some people with OCD may need a higher dose, up to 60 mg/day. Fluoxetine has a half-life of more than 80 hours, which means that it remains in the body for weeks after someone stops taking it. This long half-life also means that some people can take the medication only two or three times a week, rather than daily.

  Fluoxetine, like most of the SSRIs, is now available in generic form. This means it has gone from one of the more expensive antidepressants to one of the least expensive.
- *Citalopram (Celexa)* is typically used between 20 and 40 mg/day. It is one of the "cleaner" SSRIs, meaning that it is very selective for serotonin, and it tends to have fewer drug–drug interactions that can dangerously increase the serum level of other medications.
- *Escitalopram (Lexapro)* is the "stereoisomer" of citalopram. Most medications are a mixture of a "left" and "right" form of the same molecule. Just as your right and left hands are mirror opposites of each other, stereoisomers are similarly mirror opposites. In most biological systems, the left and right version of the molecule have different effects. Citalopram is the mixture of both forms of the molecule, one active and one largely inactive; escitalopram is the same molecule, but only the form that is biologically active. For complicated reasons, it takes a bit more than twice as much citalopram to equal the same effective amount of escitalopram. It probably takes 30 mg of citalopram to be as

effective as 10 mg of escitalopram. There is a major push from the pharmaceutical company that manufactures escitalopram, which is still on patent and therefore expensive, to demonstrate that it is more effective than citalopram, which is now generic and very inexpensive. I am not very impressed by these data and see no reason for most people to use an expensive medication when a much cheaper alternative seems to work just as well.

- *Sertraline (Zoloft)* is typically started at 50 mg/day and maintained between 50 and 200 mg/day. Its half-life is around 26 hours, but varies considerably from one person to the next. Sertraline is another very "clean" SSRI; all SSRIs can raise the serum level of other medications, but sertralive may do this a bit less than some of the others.

- *Paroxetine (Paxil)* is typically prescribed at 20 mg/day, with a range of 10–50 mg/day. Paroxetine has somewhat more effect on other non-serotonin receptors than the other SSRIs; that is, it is less selective than the others. It has been suggested that side effects of paroxetine include a lower incidence of nervousness and sleep problems than the other SSRIs. On the other hand, it causes more weight gain, more dry mouth and constipation, and more sedation than the other SSRIs. There is also concern that it may have more effect on a developing fetus when used by pregnant women.

- *Fluvoxamine (Luvox)* has been approved for use (along with clomipramine) for the treatment of OCD. It is usually started at 50 mg before bedtime, with a normal dose range of 100–300 mg/day. It appears to have a somewhat different side effect profile than the other SSRIs, which makes it preferred for some patients. It usually is more sedating and less likely to cause agitation than the others. As with the other SSRIs, headaches, nausea, tiredness, and sexual problems are common side effects. It has more frequent drug–drug interactions than most of the other SSRIs.

- *Serotonin and Norepinephrine Reuptake Inhibitors (SNRIs)* block the reuptake of both serotonin and norepinephrine, thereby affecting two of the two main systems associated with depression. Some experts believe that the SNRIs may be more effective than the pure SSRIs in helping more people achieve complete remission from their depression, rather than just improvement. The data supporting this supposed advantage, however, are not very convincing. On the other hand, there are some people who do not respond to SSRIs, and trying an SNRI, with its somewhat different mechanism of action, makes a lot of sense. SNRIs are more likely than SSRIs to cause elevated blood pressure, and they may have a bit more side effects. I tend to start with an SSRI and go to an SNRI (only if needed), unless there is a history of someone in the family who has had a good response to a specific SNRI medication or neuropathic pain is part of the problem. The SNRIs are more effective than other antidepressants in the treatment of neuropathic pain, including the pain associated with diabetes.

Specifics of Use

- *Venlafaxine (Effexor)* blocks the reuptake of both sero-tonin and norepinephrine, but the norepinephrine block is clinically important only when the dose is increased above 150 mg/day. At lower doses the amount of norepinephrine block is so small as to not have much clinical effect, and at low dose venlafaxine functions just like an SSRI. Venlafax-ine is a short-acting medication with a half-life of around 5 hours (although it does have an active metabolite with a longer half-life) that is usually taken twice a day. There is an extended-release form, venlafaxine XR, than can be taken once a day.

  Venlafaxine is typically started at 37.5 mg/day for 3 days and then increased to 75 mg/day. The normal dose range is 75–225 mg/day, but some people respond better at higher doses, and up to 375 mg or even higher can be used safely. Many of the side effects are dose related. Raising the dose may make it more effective but also cause more side effects.

  Like the SSRIs, venlafaxine is generally well tolerated. It is more likely to cause blood pressure elevation than the

SSRIs, especially in doses above 225 mg/day, and it may be a bit more likely to cause nausea when it is first started.

Otherwise, venlafaxine seems to have side effects that are very similar to the SSRIs, including headache and sleep disruption, which tend to get better after a few days at any given dose, and sexual side effects, which tend to be dose related and do not get better unless the dose is lowered. Venlafaxine can also cause some dizziness in some people, especially when first started.

Venlafaxine is somewhat more dangerous than the SSRIs if taken as an overdose. In addition, it seems to cause more withdrawal problems than the other antidepressants, especially if it is stopped too quickly. Even missing venlafaxine for a day is often uncomfortable, although the withdrawal is not medically dangerous. On the other hand, some clinicians feel that it is more effective than the SSRIs, it is more helpful with certain kinds of pain, and it is different enough from the other medications that people who have not responded to an SSRI may respond well to this SNRI.

Drug–drug interactions. Fluoxetine can interfere with the metabolism of venlafaxine. If a person is switching from one to the other, time must be allowed for the first drug to leave the person before a full dose of the second drug is given. Because of its short half-life, it is acceptable to go from venlafaxine to fluoxetine. Venlafaxine leaves the body with a day after the last dose is taken. Fluoxetine, however, has a very long half-life, and a measurable serum level that lasts several weeks after the final dose is taken. As a result, when switching from fluoxetine to venlafaxine (the more common order of switching), the venlafaxine must be introduced at a low dose, and increased gradually over the course of several weeks.

- *Duloxetine (Cymbalta)* is an SNRI that affects norepinephrine reuptake as well as serotonin over its entire dose range. It is typically started at 30 mg/day, taken with food, usually in the morning. It can be increased to 60 mg/day after 3–7 days. It can be used up to 120 mg/day, but it is unclear if

120 mg is any more effective than 60 mg for most people, and it has increased risk of side effects. As with the other SNRIs, duloxetine can raise blood pressure. Nausea is more frequently a problem with duloxetine than with other similar antidepressants. This initial nausea can be decreased by taking the medication with food or by increasing the dose a bit more slowly. It has a 12-hour half-life, so it usually is taken once per day. The tablet has a special coating to prevent its being degradation by stomach acid and passing into the rest of the gastrointestinal track, where it can be absorbed. This means that the medication will not be properly absorbed if the tablet is cut or crushed.

There have recently been some reports of very rare but very serious liver failure associated with duloxetine. This drug should be used with caution in someone with preexisting liver problems or with anyone who is a heavy user of alcohol. Anyone on duloxetine should see a physician if he or she develop abdominal pain or jaundice (skin turns yellow).

- *Desvenlafaxine (Pristiq)* is a metabolite of venlafaxine that is now marketed as a medication in its own right. There is a question about whether desvenlafaxine has real advantages over venlafaxine, its older cousin, or whether it is just a way to bring out a new medication that is still on patent and still expensive to replace an older medication that is available as an inexpensive generic. Desvenlafaxine may have fewer drug–drug interactions than venlafaxine, the parent compound, and may not need the complicated titration that venlafaxine requires. It is a new medication and we know less about its use and side effects, but it seems very much like venlafaxine. There are no convincing data that desvenlafaxine is any more effective or has any fewer side effects than venlafaxine.

Side Effects

SSRIs and SNRIs tend to have very similar side effects. Both have different side effect profiles than the older, tricyclic antidepressants. As a group, the SSRIs/SNRIs are well tolerated with fewer side effects than the older antidepressants. Some people complain of nausea and headaches when the medication is first started, although these usually disappears in a few days or weeks. For most people, the SSRIs/SNRIs tend to be activating rather than sedating, and some people feel a sense of agitation or restlessness. The SSRIs/SNRIs can interfere with sleep in some people, whereas others report sedation and a sense of lethargy. Nightmares or vivid dreams are sometimes reported. Some people also feel "blunted," as though their emotional reaction is less than it was before starting medication. A sense of motor restlessness (akathisia) is also sometimes a problem, although this is much rarer than with the antipsychotics.

SSRIs/SNRIs initially tend to cause less weight gain than older antidepressants. Roughly one out of four people on SSRIs/SNRIs will gain weight over time, usually months after starting the medication. One study found an average weight gain of around 4 pounds over 24 weeks.

Sexual dysfunction, both difficulty achieving orgasm and decreased libido, is a fairly common dose-related side effect of this class of medication. This is often the biggest problem with the SSRIs/SNRIs, and often there is no good solution, other than switching the person to an antidepressant with fewer sexual side effects. At times, adding bupropion (Wellbutrin) reverses the sexual side effects caused by an SSRI or SNRI. A long list of other medications has been used, none of which is reliable, all of which have their own side effects, but all may help some people. Medications used to treat the sexual side effects of the SSRIs/SNRIs include cyproheptadine (Periactin), yohimbine (Yocon), amantadine (Symmetrel), and sildenafil (Viagra).

There is a rare risk of bleeding with all of the SSRIs/SNRIs, primarily gastrointestinal and uterine bleeding, especially in older people. There is also rare risk of hyponatremia (decreased sodium), again more common in older people. Although this side effect is rare, anyone who has recently started on an SSRI/SNRI and who complains of lethargy, delirium or nausea should have a serum sodium test just to make sure.

The SNRIs must be used with some caution in people with glaucoma (increased pressure within the eye).

Suicide is always a risk for depressed people who are beginning to come out of their depression and become activated, but there is no evidence that fluoxetine (Prozac) or other medications in this class increase this risk. SSRIs/SNRIs are much less lethal after an overdose than tricyclic antidepressants and have fewer cardiac side effects.

Drug–Drug Interactions

P450 Enzyme Inhibition
SSRIs/SNRIs can interfere with the metabolism of many common medications. Many different medications are broken apart and made harmless in the liver by a set of enzymes called the P450 system. All SSRIs/SNRIs interfere with these enzymes to varying degrees, which in turn can cause normally prescribed doses of other medications to build up to dangerous levels. To further complicate matters, different SSRIs/SNRIs interfere with different enzymes in the P450 system, which means that different SSRIs/SNRIs interact with different medications. Paroxetine (Paxil) and fluoxetine (Prozac) cause the most inhibition of the enzyme that metabolizes tricyclic antidepressants, and they have the largest potential for causing dangerous increases in serum levels when they are given along with medications such as desipramine or amitriptyline. Fluvoxamine (Luvox) interferes with the enzyme that metabolizes clozapine enough to double its blood level. Some of these interactions can be toxic.

There are more than 30 specific enzymes in the P450 system, and no one can keep all of the interactions in mind. What is important to remember is that different SSRIs/SNRIs interfere with different parts of this system, and that the serum level of many common medications can increase dramatically when the common medication is given along with an SSRI/SNRI. Most pharmacists have computer programs that can be used to check for interactions among the list of medications that a person is taking.

HIV Medications

There are important drug–drug interactions between antidepressants and many of the medications used in the treatment of HIV. For example, Norvir and Kaletra both inhibit the enzymes that are used to metabolize the tricyclic medications, fluoxetine, fluvoxamine, and venlafaxine. When taken together, the antidepressant should be used at ¼ to½ of the normal dose. Bupropion (Wellbutrin) can have even larger, potentially dangerous increases in serum level when given along with these HIV medications.

Serotonin Syndrome

Serotonin syndrome is a risk whenever different medications that affect the serotonin system are used at the same time. Some combinations are more dangerous than others. The most dangerous interaction is between an SSRI (or SNRI) and an MAOI antidepressant, although on rare occasions this syndrome can occur as an interaction with other drugs or even as a side effect of an SSRI alone. Symptoms include confusion, agitation, sweating, increased reflexes, myoclonus (sudden jerking movements), shivering, tremor, problems with coordination, fever, and diarrhea. Serotonin syndrome can also occur when SSRIs/SNRIs are taken along with a number of other medications, including dextromethorphan, a very common ingredient in cough medications.

There is some risk of serotonin syndrome when combining two different SSRIs or in using an SSRI along with an SNRI, and there is little reason to use these combinations. On the other hand, these medications can and frequently are combined with antidepressants with different mechanisms of action, such as bupropion or mirtazapine.

Drug Withdrawal

People who abruptly stop an SSRI/SNRI (and most other antidepressants) may have uncomfortable but not dangerous withdrawal symptoms for up to several days or longer. These withdrawal symptoms can include dizziness, headaches, nausea, vivid dreams, sleep problems, irritability, and paresthesias (sense of prickling or burning of the skin). These withdrawal symptoms are more common with shorter-activating medication, such as paroxetine, fluvoxamine, and venlafaxine, and much less common with sertraline and fluoxetine.

Use in Pregnancy

There are some recent data that a pregnant woman's use of an SSRI may lower birth weight and perhaps increase the risk of respiratory distress in the newborn. These possible effects seem to be linked to duration of fetal exposure to the medication, suggesting that tapering off antidepressants during the third trimester may make some sense. There is also some risk of a withdrawal syndrome if the mother is taking an antidepressant at the time of birth. The risk of maternal depression on the fetus and the newborn must be balanced against the risk from medication. This decision should be made by the woman, but my feeling is that if medication is needed to treat a serious depression, then it should continue to be used.

Selective Norepinephrine Reuptake Inhibitor (NRIs)

Atomoxetine (Strattera) is an NRI, but it does not seem to be an effective antidepressant (it is currently available for the treatment of ADHD). Reboxetine is an NRI that seems to be an effective antidepressant. It is already available in Europe, but its patent has expired, and it is unlikely that any pharmaceutical company will obtain FDA approval to market it. It is well tolerated and may work for different people than the already available medications, although some research has suggested that overall it may be less effective than standard antidepressants already in use. Roboxetine and other NRIs may be particularly effective in people who appear to be chronically tired, apathetic, and have problems with motivation; it may end up being most useful in combination with other SSRI-type antidepressants. Side effects are different from the SSRIs. Related to increased norepinephrine, the common side effects include increased sweating, blurred vision, dry mouth, and insomnia.

Antidepressants That Act Indirectly on Serotonin and Norepinephrine

A number of antidepressants also have action on the serotonin and norepinephrine system, though through indirect mechanisms. These medications may work in some people who do not respond to SSRIs. The most important difference is that these antidepressants do not commonly have sexual side effects.

Trazodone (Desyrel)

Trazodone is FDA approved as an antidepressant, but it is much more commonly used as a sleeping pill. It is effective, inexpensive, and not addictive. It is not FDA approved as a sleeping pill and there are no long-term studies of its use in sleep, but it is very commonly used for this purpose. Trazodone is sometimes prescribed to help people overcome the sleep difficulties caused by activating antidepressants such as fluoxetine (Prozac). Trazodone is a short-acting medication with a half-life of about 3½ hours. This means that most people can take it before bedtime to help them sleep and have little sedation or hangover the next day.

Specifics of use. A typical dose of trazodone for sleep is 50 or 100 mg given before bed, although a higher dose can be used safely. Trazodone will not interfere with other antidepressants that the person may also be taking. When used as an antidepressant the typical dose is up to 600 mg/day, given in divided doses throughout the day. At this dose, most people have significant problems with sedation and often weight gain.

Side effects. The most serious (but thankfully very rare) problem with trazodone is priapism (very painful, long-lasting erection of the penis), which in extreme cases has required surgery to relieve the pressure and has led to permanent impotence in a few people. Any man prescribed trazodone should be warned about this very rare side effect and instructed to stop taking the medication if he experiences any unusual or prolonged erections.

Nefazodone (Serzone)

Nefazodone is similar to trazodone but appears to be more beneficial because it has several active metabolites that are more effective antidepressants than the parent medication. It works through a somewhat different mechanism than other antidepressants. Unfortunately it can cause rare but extremely serious liver dysfunction and is now very rarely used. The risk is present only when the medication is first started, so anyone who is currently taking the medication can probably continue it with little risk.

Specifics of use. Nefazodone seems most effective at a 300–600 mg/day dose range. Because some of the metabolites have a short half-life, twice-a-day dosing is indicated. It is generally started at 50–100 mg twice per day, and then increased.

Side effects. Other than the rare but very serious risk of liver problems, nefazodone has relatively few side effects in most people. Some people report sedation, nausea, dizziness, and anticholinergic side effects, including dry mouth, constipation, and blurred vision. As with the SSRIs, patients may experience headaches and nausea. Nervousness, weight gain, and palpitations all seem less common with nefazodone than with the SSRIs. The incidence of sexual side effects is very low—much lower than with many other antidepressants. Nefazodone also has very little tendency to cause weight gain. It has some significant drug–drug interactions.

Mirtazapine

Mirtazapine (Remeron) is an antidepressant that has both serotonin and norepinephrine activity, but it works presynaptically. This is an entirely different mechanism of action than any of the other antidepressants. It can be combined with other antidepressants, including SSRIs, SNRIs, or bupropion, if one medication alone is not enough. Its effect on different receptors seems to change with a change in dose. It is often more sedating in lower doses than in higher doses, which means that people may have fewer side effects if it is started at full dose rather than gradually increased the way most medications are. Mirtazapine is effective with anxiety, especially GAD, panic disorder, and PTSD, but may be less effective than an SSRI in OCD. It is very sedating and can be useful in reversing the sleep problems common to depression; unfortunately, sedation can also be a significant side effect. It has minimal sexual side effects.

Specifics of use. Mirtazapine is typically started at 15 or 30 mg before bedtime and can be increased to 60 mg or even higher.

Side effects include sedation and increased appetite; weight gain is frequent and can be significant. The weight gain usually begins early, and if it does not start in the first 6 weeks, it probably will not happen later.

On the other hand, there are few sexual side effects with this medication. Dizziness can be an uncommon problem, especially when the medication is first started. It has relatively mild anticholinergic side effects, including dry mouth and constipation. It seems to have relatively few drug–drug interactions and seems relatively safe in overdose.

Antidepressant That Has an Indirect Effect on Dopamine

Bupropion (Wellbutrin) seems to have an effect on the dopamine system. This dopamine activity seems to explain some of this medication's unique properties. In general, it has fewer side effects and is better tolerated than most other antidepressant medications. It is an activating rather than a sedating medication, and seems to be particularly useful in people who complain of fatigue and loss of energy. Unlike other available antidepressants, it does not cause weight gain. Furthermore, it is relatively safe if taken in overdose. Other than dangerous interactions with MAOIs, it has relatively few drug-drug side effects. It has few anticholinergic side effects (dry mouth, blurred vision, constipation), causes little problem with blood pressure, and has less effect on the electrical activity of the heart.

The big advantage of bupropion is that it does not cause any sexual side effects. In fact, it can sometimes reverse the sexual side effects caused by other medications and may be given along with an SSRI to both enhance the effectiveness of the first medication while also decreasing the sexual side effects.

Specifics of use. A normal dose of bupropion is 300–400 mg/day, usually divided into three 100 mg doses. To decrease the risk of seizure, no single dose of the regular or short-acting bupropion should exceed 150 mg. It is typically started at 100 mg twice a day, and increased no sooner than every 3 days.

A sustained-acting version of bupropion SR (Wellbutrin SR) is also available. Up to 400 mg of the long-acting bupropion can be given as 200 mg twice a day, rather than taking the medication three times a day, as regular bupropion requires at that dose. The incidence of seizures is reported to be lower with the long-acting bupropion. The long-acting bupropion has lower peak levels of medication and therefore affects the dopamine system somewhat less than the standard bupropion. Some people may not respond as well to the long-acting medication, but the increased safety, increased convenience, and decreased risk make the long-acting form the choice of most people.

Finally, an extended long-acting once-a-day version is available, bupropion XL. This is most convenient and is now available as a generic medication (called Budeprion XL)

Bupropion is the only antidepressant medication that is effective in helping people stop smoking. It seems to stop the craving associated with smoking withdrawal and works best when given along with a nicotine patch and as part of a smoking cessation program. One typically sets a "stop smoking day" 7–10 days after starting bupropion. Patients participating in smoking cessation studies are started at 150 mg/day for 3 days and then increased to 150 twice a day.

Bupropion is also effective for mild to moderate ADD (attention-deficit disorder). Although it is not as effective as a stimulant for this condition, it has the advantage of few side effects and no abuse potential.

Side effects. Bupropion is activating rather than sedating. This means that it does not cause tiredness, but it also does not help with sleep. There used to be concern that it would make anxiety worse, but this does not seem to be the case. On the other hand, it is less useful than the SSRIs in treating anxiety disorders such as panic disorder or OCD. Some people report that taking bupropion is a bit like taking caffeine, and side effects can include a sense of restlessness and sometimes sleep problems. Nausea and tremors are possible but rare.

Bupropion's introduction was delayed because of a concern about the risk of seizures. While this risk is somewhat higher with bupropion than other antidepressants, it is still low if the person does not have other risks for seizure or is not taking a larger-than-recommended dose. The seizure incidence is dose related and increases significantly when the dose is increased above 450 mg/day.

TRICYCLIC ANTIDEPRESSANTS

The first widely used antidepressants, starting in the 1950s, were the "tricyclics" (having a three-ring molecular structure). They include amitriptyline (Elavil), nortriptyline (Pamelor), desipramine (Norpramin), doxepin (Sinequan), and clomipramine (Anafranil). Although newer, safer, and better tolerated antidepressants have largely replaced these older medications, they still have an important role for people who do not respond to the newer medications, and for people with migraine headaches and other kinds of pain.

The tricyclic antidepressants are at least as effective (and sometimes more effective) as any of the newer medications for treatment of depression. With the exception of clomipramine, the tricyclics are less effective in the treatment of OCD and some of the other anxiety disorders. The major problem with these older medications is that they are much more dangerous, especially in overdose. A month's worth of any of these older medications is lethal if taken all at once. These older medications also make people feel "drugged" and sedated much more than the newer medications.

Specifics of Use

For anyone under 16 or over 40, or anyone who has a history of heart problems, a preliminary EKG is required before starting a tricyclic antidepressant. If there is any possibility of heart disease, a medical clearance should be obtained as well. The usual starting dose for imipramine (Tofranil) and amitriptyline (Elavil) is 50–75 mg/day for 2–3 days, although in older or medically ill people much lower initial doses can be used. If there are no serious side effects, gradually increase the dose to 150–300 mg/day. It takes from 5 days to 3 weeks for these medications to become effective, and a reasonable clinical trial is at least 3 weeks of medication in doses above 150 mg/day. After the dose is stabilized, most or all of the medication can be given right before bedtime to minimize the sedative and other side effects and to ensure a good night's sleep.

It is now possible to determine how much medication is actually present in the body. One person may have 10 times the serum level of another person taking the same daily dose of medication. For some medications, such as nortriptyline, there appears to be a "therapeutic window"; that is, serum levels within a certain range (50–150 mg/ml) are more effective than levels below or above this range. For other antidepressants, lower levels seem ineffective whereas higher levels are, except for their higher side effects, okay. Although we now can measure the serum levels of most antidepressants, there still is too little research for us to fully understand what the serum levels mean and how much medication is too much.

Some antidepressants such as fluoxetine (Prozac) can interfere with the metabolism of many other medications, including tricyclic antidepressants. This means that if a medication like fluoxetine is prescribed along with a tricyclic such as desipramine, a normal dose of desipramine can rapidly increase to a dangerous serum level. The same thing can happen if a patient is rapidly switched from fluoxetine to desipramine.

Side Effects

Because tricyclic antidepressants are all extremely dangerous when taken as an overdose, a severely depressed, potentially suicidal client should not be given more than a week's supply of these antidepressants without careful consideration. All of the newer antidepressants are much safer if taken as an overdose.

The tricyclic antidepressants potentiate the effect of alcohol, and a few drinks may make a person taking these medications more intoxicated than he or she would normally get. In addition, alcohol increases the lethality of antidepressants, and a normally nonlethal overdose may become lethal if combined with alcohol.

Anticholinergic side effects are common. All the traditional, tricyclic antidepressants block the action of acetylcholine and produce the kind of autonomic side effects (that is, side effects related to the involuntary part of the nervous system responsible for basic system regulation) typical of other anticholinergic medications. These include dry mouth, blurred vision, constipation, and, in rare cases, urinary retention, heart palpitations or tachycardia (speeding pulse), and increased sweating. These medications can, on rare occasions, aggravate certain kinds of glaucoma (increased pressure in the eyeball) and eye pain, which can be helped by special eyedrops.

Anticholinergic medications can also cause confusion and delirium, especially in elderly people who may be taking a number of different medications with anticholinergic side effects.

Cardiovascular side effects include orthostatic hypotension (drop in blood pressure when standing up), increased pulse, and EKG changes. The most serious of these side effects are sudden cardiac arrhythmias (irregularities of the heart beat) and heart block (when the electrical impulses cannot spread through the heart normally). Sudden death has been reported, but it is extremely rare. Overall, the effects on the heart are very complicated and not all bad. The tricyclic antidepressants (e.g., amitriptyline, desipramine) act on the heart very much like quinidine, a medication used to stabilize certain kinds of heart rhythm irregularities. In fact, a person with heart problems who normally requires quinidine or a similar medications used to treat heart arrhythmias can often reduce or eliminate his or her dose if he or she begins taking one of these antidepressants.

Neurological complications are fairly rare, though there is a very small risk of grand mal seizures with this class of medications. Other side effects of the tricyclics include drowsiness, slurred speech, and hand tremor. Like any other medication with anticholinergic properties, these medications can also cause confusion or even delirium that may be difficult to distinguish from a psychotic episode.

Weight gain is a potential problem with all of the tricyclic and MAOI antidepressants as well as the SSRIs and SNRIs. This potential for weight gain varies from one medication to another, and none of these medications typically cause the large weight gain seen in some of the antipsychotic medications.

Many antidepressants, including the tricyclics, can cause decreased libido and impotence. They can also block menstrual periods, although this seems less common. Decreasing the dose or switching antidepressants may solve these problems.

All antidepressant medications can trigger a manic episode in some susceptible people, but this may be more likely with the tricyclics than with the newer antidepressants. In addition, some people with schizophrenia are reported to become more disorganized or more paranoid when taking antidepressants. These medications can also cause some people to start "rapid cycling"—that is, to experience rapid mood swings more than once a month.

Various allergies can also occur, and any person on any medication who reports a new rash should have it investigated. Also, as with the antipsychotic medications, agranulocytosis (sudden block in white blood cell production) has been reported. If a person on one of these medications develops a sore throat, sudden chills, or fever, a physician should be alerted and a complete blood count (*CBC*) should be drawn immediately.

Abrupt withdrawal of these medications sometimes produces nausea, vomiting, abdominal cramps, diarrhea, chills, insomnia, and anxiety lasting 3–5 days. This withdrawal is not medically dangerous but can be uncomfortable. These medications usually should be withdrawn gradually over several weeks or even longer, especially if the person has been taking a medication for some time.

MONOAMINE OXIDASE INHIBITORS (MAOIS)

MAOIs block the action of the enzyme that deactivates neurotransmitters with a single amine group; hence their name *mono* (one) amine oxidase inhibitors. They can be taken as a pill—tranylcypromine (Parnate) and phenelzine (Nardil)—or as a daily patch. While the mechanism of action and the effectiveness of the medication is the same whether taken by pill or by patch, the interaction between food and the medication is very different; the daily patch avoids many of the dangerous medication–food interactions that are a problem with this class of medications. They have always been used more commonly in England, but they have been used more frequently in the United States over the past few years with the introduction of a selegiline patch.

Some people who have not responded to other medications respond to MAOIs, and they seem to be particularly useful in people with "atypical depression." These people often have problems with anxiety and agoraphobic symptoms, may have weight gain instead of the more common weight loss, and may sleep too much instead of too little. Some researchers suggest that people with "hysteroid dysphoria," a vague constellation of symptoms including marked sensitivity to rejection, which never made it into an official diagnostic system, may respond specifically to MAOIs. Others feel that people with bulimia and agoraphobia may respond better to these medications than to traditional antidepressants.

Specifics of Use

- Tranylcypromine is usually started at 10 mg two or three times a day, increasing after a week as needed. The typical dose of tranylcypromine is 40–60 mg/day, but higher doses are sometimes required.

- Phenelzine is started at 15 mg two or three times a day, with a normal dose range between 45 and 90 mg/day.

Hypertensive Crisis: Tyramine-Containing
Foods and Serotonin Syndrome

Often higher doses of these medications are more effective than lower doses, but the side effects also mount with the increasing dose, as does the risk of interactions with other medications or with tyramine-containing food. The biggest concern with oral MAO inhibitors is a hypertensive crisis (very rapid, very high, and dangerous elevation of blood pressure). This reaction is caused by an interaction between the MAOI and foods containing tyramine, or between the MAOI and medications can lead to the serotonin syndrome. There is also concern that medications that have sympathomimetic effects (that is, effects on the sympathetic nervous system) may be a problem, although this is not entirely clear. The MAOIs work by interfering with the enzyme that breaks apart certain neurotransmitters. This same enzyme also breaks apart tyramine, an amino acid that naturally occurs in certain foods. Tyramine can cause a dramatic and dangerous spike in blood pressure if it is allowed to accumulate. Normally it is so rapidly deactivated that dangerous levels never accumulate, no matter how much tyramine-containing food a person eats. Because the MAOI keeps this tyramine from being deactivated, it can rapidly accumulate to high levels and cause the dangerous increase in blood pressure.

The symptoms of a hypertensive crisis include a severe headache, heart palpitations, nausea and vomiting, unexplained nosebleed, and chest pain. A blood pressure check can quickly determine whether or not there is a problem. Such crises are rare, especially if a person is compliant with the food restrictions, but they can potentially lead to strokes and other catastrophes.

Foods that have high levels of tyramine that should be avoided include:
- Aged cheeses (and very smelly cheeses)
- Smoked or pickled fish
- Broad beans (fava beans)

- Concentrated yeast extract (e.g., Marmite, Vegemite and other concentrated yeast products), soy sauce, tofu
- Tap beer (bottled beer does not seem to be a problem)
- Sauerkraut
- Sausage, salami, and other aged meat
- Dried, salted fish
- Any food that is not fresh

MAOI Patch

When an MAOI is absorbed through the skin via a patch, it goes directly from the skin into the bloodstream and then into the brain. It does not go through the gastrointestinal (GI) tract or the liver. This means that a much lower level of medication is needed to get an effective amount into the brain, and the monoamine oxidase that is in the GI tract is not affected. Tyramine can build up only when the monoamine oxidase in the GI tract is blocked. Because the patch does not inhibit monoamine in the gut (or does so far less than the pills), there is much less risk of a problem if a food containing tyramine is eaten. As the dose of the patch increases, some of the MAOI in the gut is inhibited, and there is some risk of interactions with tyramine-containing food, but the risk is much lower than when the medication is taken in pill form.

Note that the patch does not change the problem of dangerous interactions with other medications, but only the interactions with food.

- Selegiline patch (Emsam) is usually started 6 mg patch/day. Replace the patch with a new one every 24 hours. Dose can be increased to 9 or 12 mg patch, but there is more concern about tyramine-containing food as the dose is increased.

Interactions with other Medications

MAOIs interact with a large number of other medications, often in dangerous ways. For example, extremely dangerous interactions occur when meperidine (Demerol) is taken by someone also taking an MAOI. Dextromethorphan, found in many over-the-counter cough medications, is also dangerous. In fact, many nonprescription cold, allergy, and asthma medications can cause a hypertensive reaction, as can stimulants such as amphetamines and cocaine. A potentially fatal "serotonin reaction" can occur when MAOIs are given along with SSRIs and other antidepressants that affect serotonin. Because fluoxetine (Prozac) has a long half-life, a person should not take an MAOI until he or she has been off fluoxetine for at least 5 weeks.

People taking MAOIs are strongly advised to check with their doctor or pharmacist about medication interactions before taking any other medication, whether prescribed or over-the-counter. In addition, people taking MAOIs should let all treating physicians, dentists, and other health care providers know exactly what medications they are taking. Some form of emergency notification, such as a card in their wallet or I.D. bracelet, is also a useful precaution.

Side Effects

- *MAOIs can cause orthostatic hypotension* (drop in blood pressure when client standing quickly). This can cause temporary dizziness or even fainting.
- *MAOIs are activating rather than sedating medications for most people.* This is often an advantage, since these medications usually do not cause the sedation that is common with other antidepressants, but this activating effect can interfere with sleep. Most people prefer to take these medications early in the day rather than at night, when tricyclics are usually taken. At times it is useful to give low-dose trazodone at night if sleep disturbance is a significant problem. Some people do feel sedated from the MAOIs, and feeling lethargic a few hours after taking the medication is not uncommon.
- *Other side effects are usually less common and less of a problem.* Constipation or diarrhea is sometimes reported, as is dry mouth, transient impotence, skin rash, and blurred vision, despite the fact that MAOIs are not anticholinergic. Serious liver toxicity is rare but has been reported with phenelzine (Nardil).
- *As with other antidepressants, problems can occur if an MAOI*

is stopped abruptly. Withdrawal symptoms include confusion, irritability, agitation, depression, and manic symptoms.

VITAMIN SUPPLEMENT: FOLIC ACID AND L-METHYFOLATE (DEPLIN)

Folic acid (folate) is one of the essential B complex vitamins. Humans cannot make folic acid, so it must be absorbed from food. Low folic acid levels can lead to a variety of problems, including anemia, tiredness, and serious birth defects. L-methyfolate, which is derived from folic acid, is an important regulator in the synthesis of serotonin, norepinephrine, and dopamine, the three neurotransmitters that are involved in depression. There are some data that low levels of folic acid in the blood may predispose a person to depression, and that giving folic acid may increase the effectiveness of antidepressants in people who have not responded well to antidepressants alone. Folic acid is both very inexpensive and very low in risk.

Folic acid cannot cross the blood–brain barrier until it is transformed into L-methyfolate. There ae some data indicating that some people may have a genetic deficit that interferes with folate crossing the blood–brain barrier. Even for people without this genetic deficit, there is some suggestion that the level of L-methyfolate in the brain is higher if this form of folate is taken rather than generic folic acid.

L-methyfolate is now available as Deplin, a prescription medication. Deplin is much more expensive than generic folic acid. There is an open question about whether to use inexpensive folic acid or the much more expensive prescription L-methyfolate. I think that it makes sense for anyone who is depressed to consider taking folic acid or a vitamin that contains folic acid. There are data that taking folic acid may decrease some kinds of birth defects, and any women who could possibly become pregnant should be taking some form of folic acid just in case a pregnancy did ensue. If a person continues to feel depressed after trying several antidepressants

aking folic acid, it may be worthwhile to see if Deplin
des any additional help.

DECIDING WHICH ANTIDEPRESSANT TO USE

All of the antidepressants currently available seem equally effective, although a particular medication may be dramatically more
effective than another for a particular individual. Unfortunately,
there is no way to be certain about which medication will work
for which client. Physicians are often inclined to select certain
antidepressants because they are familiar with them. It is reasonable to select the medication with a side effect profile that is likely
to be least troublesome to the particular client. The main side
effects to consider in choosing a medication are degree of sedation, degree of anticholinergic activity, cardiovascular side effects
(including orthostatic hypotension), and sexual side effects. For
example, citalopram has not anticholinergic side effects (dry
mouth, blurred vision, urinary retention, etc.). This might be a
good medication for people who have had problems with constipation or blurred vision. It can cause weight gain, however. It
also commonly causes some degree of sexual dysfunction. Citalopram is generally not sedating, which most people consider an
advantage. Doxepin (Sinequan), on the other hand, is very sedating, and for people with insomnia this medication's sedative side
effect might be useful if there is little risk of overdose. If sexual
side effects are a concern, bupropion (Wellbutrin) or nefazodone
(Serzone) might be the best choice.

When the first antidepressant does not work and a second
medication is being considered, it makes sense to choose one that
is as different as possible from the first, although there are few
hard data to support this theory. All six classes of antidepressants
(SSRIs/SNRIs/NRIs, mirtazapine, bupropion, tricyclics, MAOIs,
nefazodone) have somewhat different mechanisms of action.
Occasionally, a client will respond to one medication and not
another, even though the medications are of the same type.

A number of augmentation strategies are worth trying when a
single antidepressant medici0on is not effective. The most com-

mon strategy is switching to another antidepressant or adding a second antidepressant with a different mechanism of action. Other strategies include adding a mood stabilizer such as lithium or one of the second-generation antipsychotic medications to the antidepressant. Adding folic acid makes sense, either in the inexpensive generic form or as the more expensive L-methyfolate. Still other augmentation strategies include the use of thyroid hormone even when there appears to be normal thyroid function.

Table 5.1 summarizes the side effects of commonly prescribed antidepressant medications.

Electroconvulsive Therapy (ECT)

ECT is has a negative reputation, but modern ECT, when used in people with serious depression, is safe, fast, and can be life-saving. ECT is often effective when even medication is not.

Psychotherapy:

It may seem very odd to include psychotherapy as way to change brain chemistry, but there is increasing research data to support it. Psychotherapy is the process of learning new skills and behaviors that can help to change our feelings and how well we can cope with the world. There are many different types of psychotherapies and many different areas of potential focus. For example, we can identify specific triggers that tend to cause us to get angry, and then figure out new ways to deal with these anger-inducing situations when they arise. We can identify assumptions that we often rely on, and then examine these assumptions to see if they are really accurate. This can help us to feel and behave differently in situations that have previously been problematic.

A specific psychotherapeutic approach that is particularly useful in the treatment of depression is called cognitive–behavioral therapy, or CBT. It is virtually impossible to consciously our emotions, and to simply decide to feel happier or less anxious. However, we can learn what factors cause those emotions, and thus learn to avoid or replace those factors. This is the key idea behind CBT. If we think about some pleasant event, we tend to feel happy. If we

TABLE 5.1. Side Effects of Common Antidepressant Medications

	Sedation	Insomnia	Dry Mouth	Constipation	Blood Pressure Drop	GI Distress	Weight Gain	Sexual Problems
Amitriptyline	+++	+	+++	+	+	+	+++	+
Bupropion	0	+	+	+	0	0	0	0
Citalopram	+	+	+	0	0	0	+	++
Fluoxetine	+	+	+	0	+	+	0 to +	+++
Duloxetine	+	+	+	+	+	+	0	+++
Fluvoxamine	+	+	+	+	0	0	+	+++
Mirtazapine	+++	0	+++	+	0	0	+++	0
Nortriptyline	++	0 to +	+	+	0 to +	0 to +	+	0 to +
Paroxetine	+	+	+	+	+	+	++	+++
Sertraline	+	+	+	0	+	+	0 to +	+++
Venlafaxine	+	+	+	+	+	+	+++	+++

think about a terrible event in our past, we become depressed. Our fluctuating emotions are caused by changes in brain chemistry. Just as a medication or drug can change our mood, our mood and our thinking can change our brain chemistry.

EXERCISE

Regular exercise, especially aerobic forms of exercise 3–4 times/week, has been demonstrated in a number of studies to improve mild to moderate depression. There are many reasons why exercise might help. The increased activity and the general sense of physical well-being that follows are probably important, but the specific mechanism in depression is connected with an increased release of endorphins. These trigger some of the same reward circuits that are stimulated by morphine and may explain some of the "addictive" quality of running and other aerobic exercise. I can almost guarantee that a person who is depressed will feel better if he or she engages in regular exercise. The problem is in getting someone who is depressed to do it.

LIGHTS FOR SADS (SEASONAL AFFECTIVE DISORDER)

Our brain is very sensitive to the length of the day, or more specifically to the length of the time that we are in light. In the winter, depending on our climate, the photoperiod—or the length of time when there is daylight—shortens. Those of us who live in more northern climates are well aware of this. Many people get more sluggish and "down" in the winter and feel better in the summer. Although this can be a reaction to either the cold or to decreased activity, there are good data that it is most often connected to the shortened photoperiod. Many of us tend to spend much more time indoors in the winter, which exacerbates the effects of a shortened photoperiod. Even a very brightly lit room has much less light intensity than being outside, even on a very overcast day.

Lights are used to treat SADS, very special intense lights that are filtered to remove harmful ultraviolet effects, can significantly help increase the mood of someone with SADS when used regularly in the morning. It is important to get a clear pattern of the timing of the depression before rushing into this diagnosis. Even people who do not meet formal criteria for SADS but who find themselves feeling more down in the winter might find some benefits from the regular use of these lights. Note that it is very hard to get enough light intensity from regular lighting to help very much. If you are going to use lights to treat SADS, the use of special lights is necessary. As with any effective treatment for depression, there is a very small risk of precipitating a manic episode in someone who is very susceptible. SADS lights seem most effective when used for 30–60 minutes in the morning.

STRATEGIES

If the first antidepressant does not work or does not work completely, try the following process (what to try in what order needs to be individualized for each person):
- Screen for substance use, external stressors, medical illness.
- Ask if the person is taking the medication consistently.
- Consider psychotherapy; rethink focus of therapy.
- Encourage regular exercise.
- Ensure that the person is sleeping.
  - Consider use of trazodone or other sleeping medication.
- Add an antidepressant medication with a different mechanism of action.
  - Add bupropion to an SSRI or SNRI.
  - Add mirtazapine to an SSRI or SNRI.
- Switch to another antidepressant.
  - Another SSRI, SNRI, or newer-generation medication.
  - Consider tricyclic antidepressant.
  - Consider MAOI, either by pill or daily patch.
- Add folic acid or L-methyfolate.
- Add low dose of second-generation antipsychotic medication.
- Add lithium or valproic acid to the antidepressant.
- Add low-dose thyroid hormone (T_3 or T_4).
- Add buspirone.
- Add low-dose stimulant (amphetamine or methylphenidate).

6

Mood-Stabilizing Medications

The first effective mood stabilizer was lithium. Initially used in 1949, it was the first modern "wonder drug" in psychiatry. In addition to lithium, a number of medications initially developed to control seizures are now commonly used as mood stabilizers. Valproic acid (Depakote) and carbamazepine (Tegretol) are considered, along with lithium, to be "first-line" mood stabilizers. They can help to abort a manic episode and can decrease both the frequency and severity of future manic episodes. These traditional mood stabilizers tend to be much more effective in helping to control the "ups" or the manic part of the illness, and less effective in helping with the depression that is part of bipolar disorder.

A number of other anticonvulsants have been used as mood stabilizers, but much of this use has very little research support. Some of these anticonvulsants do have research support for other uses, such as gabapentin (Neurontin) for anxiety and pain control, and topiramate (Topamax) for the treatment of alcohol abuse and impulse control problems.

The second-generation antipsychotic medications are also effective mood stabilizers, even for people who have no psychotic symptoms. They are called "antipsychotic" because their initial use was for control of psychotic symptoms, but they could just as well have been called "mood stabilizers" if that use had been discovered first. For some people, these second-generation antipsychotic medications may be more effective or have fewer side effects than the more traditional mood-stabilizing medications. All of the second-generation antipsychotic medications are effective both in treating an acute manic episode and in helping to prevent the next manic episode. They also seem useful in the treatment of bipolar depression. At this time, it is not clear if they are all equally effective for the treatment of bipolar depression, or whether some of them may be more effective for treating this end of the bipolar swing.

Mood stabilizers are not "uppers" or "downers" or simple antidepressants. They stabilize both the highs and the lows of some people with mood swings, although some tend to be more effective with the "ups," and others are more effective against the "downs." Mood swings do not always disappear, but they often become less frequent and less severe. Classic bipolar disorder, defined by mood swings occurring less than twice a year, generally responds better to medication than does the rapid cycling type (more than four major mood swings a year), the mixed state type (elements of both mania and depression present at the same time), or other more atypical mood disorders.

As noted, the same medication than helps control an acute manic episode will also help to prevent the next manic episode—although there are exceptions to this rule of thumb. For example, a first-generation antipsychotic medication such as haloperidol or a benzodiazepine such as lorazepam can help a person who is acutely manic or hypomanic get back in control. However, neither of these medications are commonly used long-term for maintenance to prevent the next manic episode.

A major issue involves when to consider use of a medication. If a person has had several severe manic episodes, the likelihood of another episode is very high. If the previous manic episodes have caused major life problems, then it makes a lot of sense to use a medication that can decrease the risk of another such episode. In addition, there is increasing concern that each manic episode may increase the chance of having another episode. There is a tendency for people with untreated bipolar disorder to have more frequent episodes over time. For a person with a clearly diagnosed bipolar disorder, maintenance treatment with a mood stabilizer is highly likely to increase the his or her stability and lead to an improved quality of life over the long term.

Many people have mood swings that are less severe or less clear-cut than full mania. Indeed, less severe mood swings of one sort or another are very common. Some of these can cause significant life problems but are not so severe as to meet criteria for bipolar I or even bipolar II disorder. People can learn to control these mood swings in many ways. Cognitive–behavioral therapy, consistent structure in daily life, and a regular sleep pattern can all help. Mood-stabilizing medications can also help, but they all come with some risks and side effects. As always, the potential benefits of medication must be weighed and balanced by the risks and burden of the medication. How big a problem is the mood instability causing in this person's life? What else has already been tried? The decision regarding the use of medication should come out of a discussion between the prescriber and the person with the problem. Encouraging the person to bring a friend or family member can be a way of bringing another perspective into this conversation.

TERMINOLOGY

Manic–depressive disorder and *bipolar disorder* are different names for the same condition. When people are manic, they typically have grandiose thoughts, are very energetic, need very little sleep, talk very rapidly, and spend money recklessly or engage in other impulsive behavior. They are often very irritable and generally are thinking so fast that they have trouble functioning in normal activities. Some, but not all, people with mania find it enjoyable to feel that smart or that important or to think that fast. For other people, there is so much irritability or paranoia connected to the mania that it is a very distressing experience.

Hypomania is less than full mania. People who are hypomanic are less out of control, and although they may be thinking and talking rapidly, they are generally better able to function at work and at home. *Bipolar I* refers to a full manic episode, with or without a history of depression. *Bipolar II* refers to a hypomanic episode—that is, one not as severe as full mania. People in a full manic episode may have psychotic symptoms, including hallucinations and delusions, but these resolve when the mania improves. If a person continues to have psychotic symptoms after the manic symptoms have subsided, then the appropriate diagnosis is *schizoaffective disorder*. In the midst of a manic episode with psychotic symptoms, it can be extremely difficult to determine if the person has schizophrenia, mania, or schizoaffective disorder.

LITHIUM (LITHIUM CARBONATE)

The common form of lithium used in psychiatry is lithium carbonate. Lithobid, Eskalith, and Eskalith CR are brand names of lithium that are packaged so that it is absorbed somewhat more slowly, and therefore may produce fewer gastrointestinal side effects, especially less nausea.

Indications for Use

The most common indication for the use of lithium is as a mood stabilizer in the treatment of bipolar or schizoaffective disorder, or other kinds of cyclic mood disorders. It may also augment the effectiveness of an antidepressant in treatment-resistant depression. It may also help some people who experience rage reactions (uncontrollable outbursts of anger).

Bipolar I, Bipolar II, and Schizoaffective Disorders

Lithium is one of the medications of choice for helping to control the mood swings in someone who has a manic–depressive or bipolar illness. It tends to be used much more in Europe; its use in the United States has fallen off despite its effectiveness. Lithium has been shown to decrease the risk of suicide in people with bipolar disorder (the only other medication shown to decrease risk is clozapine, when used to treat schizophrenia). Lithium decreases the frequency and severity of manic episodes, but it does not necessarily eliminate them in all people. It is also useful in aborting an acute manic episode and is often used in combination with an antipsychotic medication. Lithium is useful in the mood swings associated with schizoaffective disorder and even in some people with schizophrenia who are agitated, aggressive, or displaying other manic-like symptoms. Lithium is also helpful in preventing the depressive side of manic–depressive disease.

A family history of bipolar disorder, depression, or suicide increases the probability that a person will respond to lithium. A person who reports experiencing, for example, depressions and "highs," bouts of excessive spending, or frequent and impulsive marriages should be considered as possibly having periods of mania.

Some people with a diagnosis of schizophrenia also respond to lithium. It may be that the diagnosis is incorrect and the person is really bipolar. It also appears that lithium can be useful in augmenting antipsychotic medication in people with schizophrenia. It makes sense to seriously consider a trial of lithium for someone with schizophrenia who is not responding well to more traditional therapy and who is talks rapidly and is irritable, angry, or aggressive—all of which are affective symptoms. Whenever a medication is first begun, and especially when initiating such trials, it is important to remember that they are just that—*trials*. The medication should be started and continued for a specified period of time, usually 4–6 weeks, and target symptoms that were previously identified should be used to assess whether the medication is helping.

Augmenting Antidepressants in People
with Treatment-Resistant Depression

Combining lithium and antidepressants may be effective for people who have not responded to antidepressants alone. A person who has experienced no improvement with an antidepressant alone may begin to respond when lithium is added, and a person who has had a partial response to an antidepressant may have a better response. Lithium can be safely combined with virtually all of the common antidepressant medications. There are studies showing that it can help augment the antidepressant effect of both the older tricyclic-type medications as well as SSRIs. It requires blood tests to monitor serum levels and can have bothersome side effects, however. It can also be cumbersome to use. On the other hand, for some people it can be lead to a much better treatment response. When used to augment an antidepressant, lithium carbonate is usually started at 300 mg once or twice a day and increased after a week.

Treatment of Other Cyclic Mood Disorders

Many people with borderline and other personality diagnose show marked and, at times, rapid mood changes from sad to elated and back to sad again. These mood fluctuations may not be "big enough" to meet criteria for bipolar disorder, but along with the other problems of personality disorders, they can still be a major problem for the person experiencing them. For some people, lithium or another mood stabilizer can help decrease the number and intensity of these mood fluctuations.

Anger Dyscontrol

Lithium also has been effective in some people with explosive, uncontrollable "hair-trigger"-type anger outbursts. Lithium does not help the person who is chronically angry, however. Rather, there is a specific group of people who say that when they do get angry, they lose all control and act without having the time to consider the consequences. They identify these angry outbursts as a problem. Lithium can give the person a bit more time to think about things before exploding.

Laboratory Monitoring

The most common guideline suggests that a serum BUN (blood urea nitrogen) and serum creatinine should be obtained before starting lithium to determine that the person's kidneys are working properly. Lithium is excreted by the kidneys, and if they are not working well, the lithium can build up rapidly to toxic levels. If getting a blood test is difficult and the person is healthy, I may wait to get basic kidney tests until the first lithium serum level, usually 5–7 days after starting the lithium. An initial blood test will be needed at this point to measure the amount of lithium in the person's blood, and obtaining the kidney tests at the same time avoids a need for a separate blood draw. There is some risk in this method, but it is very small. It is unlikely that a person will develop toxic kidney problems on an initially low dose of lithium in this 5 to 7-day period, and decreasing the need for blood draws increases the likelihood that the person will stay on the lithium.

Some experts suggest an EKG but, unless there is concern about heart disease, it is unnecessary. Some experts suggest a creatinine clearance test as well, but this requires collecting all of a person's urine over 24 hours, which is cumbersome, expensive, and usually impossible outside of a hospital. Following serum creatinine (which is a simple blood test) over the course of lithium therapy is a reasonably safe way to detect early kidney damage. A yearly urinalysis may give some information about the kidneys' ability to concentrate urine, but this simple test is not part of most protocols. Though there is concern about lithium and kidney damage, such damage is rare.

Lithium can decrease the production of thyroid hormone. Such a condition is easily treatable by replacing the thyroid hormone, but people should be aware of the symptoms of decreased thyroid activity (hypothyroid). A person on lithium who complains of tiredness, weight gain, intolerance to cold, or dry skin or dry hair should get a TSH test (a simple, inexpensive blood test) to assess thyroid function. Some guidelines suggest a yearly test for thyroid function, although I prefer to keep a high index of suspicion and get a TSH when symptoms suggest it is indicated. Hypothyroidism often starts very gradually, typically years after starting lithium. This makes it is easy to miss the early signs of decreased thyroid function, and often symptoms have been present for some time before hypothyroidism is diagnosed.

Specifics of Use

Start lithium by giving 600–900 mg/day in divided doses. Increase the dose as needed to maintain a desired serum level. A repeat lithium level is recommended 5–7 days after any dose change. Lithium carbonate usually comes in 300 mg capsules, so a typical dose is two to three capsules a day. Lithium used to be given two or three times a day because of concern of toxicity and side effects. Most people, once they are on a stable dose of the medication, do well taking the entire dose of lithium at one time. Taking lithium with food tends to decrease its gastrointestinal side effects.

Follow with serum lithium levels and adjust the dose so that the lithium level in the blood is 0.6–1.2 mEq/l (milliequivalents per liter, a measure of concentration). Textbooks used to suggest that lithium levels be 0.8–1.2 mEq/l. People with bipolar disorder will have less risk of relapse if their lithium level is kept between 0.8 and 1.2 mEq/l, and somewhat more risk of relapse if their level is allowed to drop to the 0.4–0.6 mEq/l range. Unfortunately, they also have poorer compliance and more side effects at the higher levels. Although there is some increased risk of relapse at the lower dose, for some people, depending on the seriousness of their disease and severity of side effects, the decrease in side effects may make this risk worthwhile. Most people require 600–1800 mg/day to maintain their serum lithium level within this therapeutic range. Older people and those with brain damage generally require less lithium and may become toxic on normal doses.

As a person ends a manic episode, less medication may be needed to maintain the same serum medication level. People who have had a stable lithium level while manic may become toxic if they continue to take the same amount of lithium after they calm down. Conversely, people going into a manic episode frequently need to increase their daily lithium dose to maintain a therapeutic serum lithium level.

When lithium is being used to augment the effectiveness of an antidepressant rather than for bipolar disorder, a lower serum lithium level, on the order of 0.5 mEq/l, may be sufficient and is usually more comfortable.

After a person seems stable on a given dose of lithium, blood levels should be measured at least every 6 months. Blood levels change during the day, peaking several hours after the person takes a dose and dropping slowly until the next dose. It is important, therefore, to standardize when the blood sample is drawn. A serum level of 0.6 mEq/l 12 hours after a dose means something different from the same level 24 hours after a dose. Standard serum levels should always be drawn as close as possible to 12 hours after a normal dose of medication is taken. A person receiving divided doses of lithium should have his or her lithium level checked before taking the morning dose, which should be about 12 hours after the evening dose was taken.

Side Effects

Lithium has a number of uncomfortable side effects that may make people reluctant to take it. With appropriate monitoring, it is generally safe, although long-term effects on the kidneys, and risk of birth defects, are common.

Common, Uncomfortable Side Effects

The most common side effect of lithium is a fine tremor of the hands that usually begins during the first few days of treatment. Nausea, vomiting, and even some mild abdominal pain are common initially but usually disappear in a few weeks. These side effects may be decreased by giving the medication in smaller divided doses, or giving it along with food so that absorption is slowed. Some weight gain is common, although it is not as frequent or as big as occurs with valproic acid (Depakote) or some other medications. A metallic taste can be a problem for some people. Lithium can also cause increased thirst and frequent urination, and it interferes with the ability of the kidneys to concentrate urine; this means that lithium causes a person to put out a larger volume of more dilute urine. Although lithium can affect the heart and cause minor changes in a person's EKGs, this is rarely a serious problem. Finally, lithium can cause some people to feel as though their thinking is a bit fuzzy or slowed down. People report that at times they feel less creative or a bit blunted in how they emotionally react to things.

Toxic Side Effects

There is only a small difference in the serum lithium level that is effective and the level that begins to cause toxic or dangerous side effects. These toxic side effects, which can look initially like an exaggeration of the common, nontoxic side effects, include thirst, decreased appetite, vomiting, and diarrhea. However, these can progress to confusion, coarse tremor, muscle twitching, and slurred speech. In extreme cases, the person appears drunk and has muscle twitches, nystagmus (small jerks of the eye), hyperreflexia (increased reflexes), seizures, stupor, and eventually coma. The neurological symptoms in such cases may be present in only one side of the body or may be more severe on one side than they are on the other.

If a person taking lithium develops diarrhea or nausea, lithium intoxication should be considered and serum lithium levels obtained.

Long-Term Effect on the Kidneys

Lithium is excreted by the kidneys. Severe kidney disease (determined by BUN and serum creatinine tests) can interfere with this normal excretion of lithium and allow a dangerous buildup of the medication in a short time. Increased fluid intake and urination are common in most people on lithium because of its direct effect on the kidneys, causing a syndrome called *nephrogenic diabetes insipides*. Although this condition is usually not dangerous, in some rare cases the increased urination may be severe enough to cause serious dehydration. These effects on the kidney rarely cause actual kidney damage and usually correct themselves when the medication is discontinued. However, a very few people on long-term lithium therapy may incur permanent, irreversible, and potentially life-threatening kidney damage. No clear information about the frequency of such damage is available, except that it seems to be rare and can be prevented by discontinuing lithium before the kidney damage gets too severe. All people on lithium should have their serum creatinine measured with a simple blood test every 6–12 months to identify early kidney damage before it can cause a significant health risk.

Treatment of Lithium Side Effects

Some of the side effects from lithium are treatable. Mild diarrhea can be treated by over-the-counter medications, such as Kaopectate. A fine *intention tremor* can be treated with a low dose of a beta-blocker (a medication that blocks the effect of epinephrine on beta receptors) such as propranolol, which is safe and easy to use. Still, using one medication to treat the side effects of another only makes sense when the tremor is causing some problem or discomfort. If frequent urination is a problem, trying to decrease fluid intake, especially in the hours before bed, may help with nighttime control. If frequent urination becomes a more serious problem for a person taking lithium, because it is either dehydrating or so frequent that it is interfering with the person's life, hydrochlorothiazide, a diuretic usually used for treatment of high blood pressure, can be used. It normally causes people to urinate more, but it works paradoxically on people suffering from increased urination because of lithium. There is some concern that hydrochlorothiazide may increase the risk of kidney damage from lithium, and it is only used when the increased urinary frequency is severe. Hydrochlorothiazide increases most people's serum lithium levels, potentially to a toxic degree. To prevent lithium toxicity, the dose of lithium is usually decreased at the same time that hydrochlorothiazide is started, and serum lithium levels are monitored carefully. Hydrochlorothiazide also causes potassium loss, which needs to be monitored and can be treated by taking orange juice or bananas.

Drug–Drug interactions

Lithium interacts with a number of commonly prescribed medications. The most common problem is a rise in the serum lithium level, at times to toxic levels, when a person initially stable on lithium begins taking an additional medication. As noted, this occurs with hydrochlorothiazide, a very common medication used for water retention and high blood pressure, and with a number of pain medications, including most of the nonsteroidal, anti-inflammatory medications such as indomethacin (Indocin), phenylbutazone (Butazolidin), and possibly ibuprofen (Motrin). Aspirin and acetaminophen (Tylenol) are safe.

Use during Pregnancy

There is evidence that lithium increases the risk of serious birth defects, especially if taken during the first 3 months of pregnancy. This risk is high enough that women who become pregnant or who are planning to become pregnant should stop taking lithium if possible.

Overdoses of Lithium

Lithium is potentially toxic when a large amount is taken as an overdose. Frequently a person overdosing on lithium will vomit it up; if the lithium is not expelled through vomiting, however, a high lithium level (above 2.5) can cause damage to the brain and kidney. Lithium overdoses must be taken very seriously. Prompt treatment can almost always avoid damage, but in some cases treatment includes the need for kidney dialysis to rapidly remove lithium from the person's blood.

DIVALPROEX SODIUM (DEPAKOTE) AND VALPROIC ACID (DEPAKENE)

Depakote is divalproex sodium, which is a compound of valproate and valproic acid. Depakene is just valproic acid. The terms *valproate*, *valproic acid*, and *divalproex sodium* are used interchangeably, and all are transformed to the exact same chemical in the body, although formally they are slightly different chemicals. When someone refers to a pill of valproate or valproic acid, he or she is simply using shorthand for the term *divalproex sodium*. *Valproic acid* is the term most commonly used for the generic version of this medication.

Indications for Use

Valproic acid was originally developed as an anticonvulsant, but it is now in widespread use as a mood stabilizer. Both valproic acid and lithium carbonate are first line medications for the treatment of bipolar illness. Lithium carbonate has been used longer, we have more information about its effectiveness, and it is much less expensive than divalproex sodium. Valproic acid can be started at a full dose essentially from the beginning and seems to work more rapidly. Both medications have their own side effects, but for many people the side effects of valproic acid may be easier to live with than those of lithium. On the other hand, the weight gain associated with valproic acid is a very big problem for many people taking it.

Relatively little research data directly compare divalproex sodium or valproic acid and lithium. My belief is that valproic acid *may* be somewhat more effective than lithium when the symptoms or illness course do not fit into a classic manic–depressive pattern. This includes people who experience rapid cycling (four or more episodes of mania or depression a year), extreme mood instability, a seizure disorder or a history of seizures, or who have any history of brain damage. Like lithium, valproic acid can also be used to increase the effectiveness of antidepressants and to treat rage reactions (uncontrollable anger).

Specifics for Use

Although some psychiatrists start valproic acid slowly and build up over several weeks, it is safe to start it more rapidly. I often start valproic acid by prescribing 500 mg tablets of divalproex sodium (Depakote) twice a day and then getting a valproic acid blood level 5 days later. It is also safe and well tolerated to begin divalproex sodium at a full dose, usually figured at 15–20 mg/kg. For example, a 220-pound (100 kg) person can be safely started on 1500–2000 mg/day in divided doses. A normal dose is 1000–2000 mg/day, but this is usually adjusted based on blood levels. Occasionally a much higher dose is required to achieve a therapeutic blood level. There is often less stomach upset if divalproex sodium is started at twice a day, but most people can take it once a day without problems after the first week or so.

The effective serum concentrations needed to prevent seizures is between 65 and 125 µg/l (micrograms per liter, a common measurement of concentrations of indications in blood serum). There is much less research on the serum level needed for valproic acid to be an effective mood stabilizer, but it seems more effective when used at the upper end of this range, usually with levels between 80–125 µg/l. It is suggested that serum levels be obtained every 6 months. It is also suggested that liver function tests be obtained every 6–12 months, although given the very low frequency of liver problems in adults, it is unclear if this is always necessary after the first 6 months.

There seems to be less gastrointestinal upset if someone is started on divalproex sodium rather than valproic acid. Both divalproex sodium and valproic acid are available as inexpensive generics. There is also an extended release form of divalproex sodium, called Depakote ER, that is not available as a generic. Some clinicians have suggested that this delayed-release form of the medication may have fewer side effects, and may even cause a bit less weight gain. These claims may turn out to be true, but so far there are few data to support these suggestions.

Use during Pregnancy

Valproic acid is associated with an increased risk of birth defects, primarily neural tube defects, when taken in the first trimester of the pregnancy. Women should be given a pregnancy test or carefully asked about the possibility of being pregnant before starting the medication.

It has been suggested that this risk of birth defects can be decreased if the women is taking extra folic acid, which is known to decrease birth defects in general. Although folic acid does not eliminate the risk of birth defects, it is inexpensive, has no side effects, and can help. Any women who has any potential of becoming pregnant should be taking folic acid or a vitamin that contains folic acid, just in case a pregnancy occurs.

Side Effects

In general, valproic acid is well tolerated. It has a bit more sedation, but perhaps a bit less restriction of creativity than is sometimes reported with lithium.

Common, Annoying, but Not Medically Dangerous Side Effects

Weight gain, which occurs in about half of the people using valproic acid, is the biggest common problem with this medication and appears to be dose related. Nausea, vomiting, and indigestion are common problems when valproic acid is first started, but these symptoms usually disappears after a week or 2. Sedation is sometimes a problem. Tremor and other motor movements are not common, but can occur. Hair loss is rare but can be a serious problem for some people. At times, the hair loss can be so severe that the medication needs to be discontinued. Hair growth may be helped with selenium and zinc mineral supplementation, and it usually resumes even if the valproic acid is continued.

Medically Dangerous Side Effects

Liver Toxicity
While valproic acid has been associated with serious liver toxicity in children, this is extremely rare in adults. If liver problems are going to occur, it will almost always be in the first 6 months of use. It is generally safe to use valproic acid with people who have hepatitis C or other liver problems, but liver function tests should be followed more frequently, depending on the seriousness of the liver problem.

Pancreatitis

There have now been reported cases of an inflammation of the pancreas connected with valproic acid. This is extremely painful and can be fatal in rare cases. The primary symptom of pancreatitis is abdominal pain. Anyone taking valproic acid who begins experiencing severe abdominal pain should be evaluated by a physician.

Polycystic Ovaries

Valproic acid has been associated with polycystic ovary disease in women of childbearing age, especially teenagers. There is debate about whether valproic acid is the direct cause of this polycystic ovary disease, or whether it is an indirect effect connected to the weight gain that is a side effect of valproic acid. It is also possible that the increased prevalence of polycystic ovary disease is not caused by the medication at all, but rather is associated with the seizure disorders that the valproic acid is often treating. Polycystic ovaries are really an endocrine problem with symptoms that include excess male pattern hair growth and decreased fertility.

Laboratory Monitoring

A screen for pregnancy should be done before starting the medication, either by taking a careful history or via a urine test. In the hospital it is recommended to get baseline labs before starting any medication, but in the community I usually wait to get a baseline WBC (white blood count) with differential and liver function tests at the time of the first blood level, usually 5–7 days after starting the medication. I may get another WBC and liver function test a month or 2 later, especially if I need another serum level, but if I have no clinical concern I may go up to 6 months for the next liver function tests, with yearly monitoring thereafter.

Drug–Drug Interactions

Valproic acid can inhibit the metabolism of other commonly used medications. This means that there can be higher serum levels of these other medications than one might expect. For example, carbamazepine levels, particularly some of its active metabolites (breakdown products), increase when it is used along with valproic acid. Valproic acid can also increase the serum levels of tricyclic antidepressants and of lamotrigine (Lamictal)—the dose of the lamotrigine is typically halved when given along with valproic acid.

CARBAMAZEPINE (TEGRETOL)

(Carbatrol and Tegretol XR are longer-acting versions of same medication.)

Indications for Use

Carbamazepine is useful for people with bipolar illness who do not respond well to lithium or valproic acid or who cannot tolerate the side effects of these other medications. One huge advantage over lithium and valproic acid is that carbamazepine does not cause weight gain. It is generally considered a "second-line" treatment and is more commonly used in Europe than in the United States. Carbamazepine can be used along with both lithium and valproic acid. It seems particularly useful for people with atypical illness or rapid cycling bipolar disorder (more than four episodes a year).

Carbamazepine is also being used in a variety of other conditions for which lithium and valproic acid have been ineffective. Some people with schizophrenia, whose ongoing affective lability makes stabilization difficult, respond well to either lithium or carbamazepine in combination with an antipsychotic medication. Some people with aggressive or violent outbursts also seem to respond to carbamazepine or one of the other mood-stabilizing medications. It was once thought that some kind of hidden seizure disorder caused these outbursts, but carbamazepine seems to be effective in people who have no evidence of any kind of seizures.

Specifics of Use

Carbamazepine is usually started at 100–200 mg twice a day, and the dose is then increased until the serum level is 5–12 µg/l.

Generally it takes around 5 days for a dose change to be fully reflected in the serum level, so it makes sense to get a serum level 5–7 days after starting the medication and after every dose change to guide the amount needed.

Carbamazepine is a short-acting medication that is usually taken twice a day, although there are now two longer-acting versions, Carbatrol and Tegretol XR. These still require twice-a-day dosing, but they maintain a steadier serum level between doses, with a lower peak serum level, which may decrease side effects in some people.

Carbamazepine induces liver enzymes. That is, over some weeks the liver increases the enzymes needed to metabolize (break down into inactive fragments) carbamazepine. As the liver becomes more efficient at metabolizing carbamazepine, the blood level will drop. This means that the carbamazepine serum level tends to drop over the first 6 weeks after it is started, even if the same dose is taken every day. (Alcohol does the same thing, which is one of the reasons seasoned drinkers can drink more without getting as drunk.)

Laboratory Monitoring

The standard recommendation is to obtain both a WBC (white blood count) and LFTs (liver function tests) before starting carbamazepine, then again in about a month, then again in 3 months, then every 6 months. In the community this is sometimes difficult to arrange. In a healthy adult I often decrease the number of required blood draws by getting the initial WBC and LFTs when I get the first carbamazepine serum level, 5–7 days after starting the medication.

People who appear confused or sedated on carbamazepine, despite having a normal serum level, have a buildup of an active metabolite of carbamazepine called 10,11 epoxide. This too can be measured if there is any clinical concern.

On rare occasions, carbamazepine can also lower serum sodium levels, so one should obtain a serum sodium level along with the other blood tests or if the person becomes confused.

Use during Pregnancy

Carbamazepine is associated with an increased risk of birth defects, especially when taken during the first trimester. Birth defects caused by carbamazepine include neural tube defects, defects in the face and skull, underdevelopment of fingernails, and developmental delay. Women should be given a pregnancy test or carefully asked about the possibility of being pregnant before starting carbamazepine.

Carbamazepine can lower the hormone level from birth control pills. As a result, birth control pills may not be effective in preventing pregnancy when taking carbamazepine.

Carbamazepine, like valproic acid and some of the other anti-convulsants, is associated with an increased rate in birth defects. As discussed in the section on valproic acid, any women who have any possibility of becoming pregnant should take folic acid or a vitamin that contains folic acid, just in case a pregnancy occurs.

Side Effects of Carbamazepine

Generally carbamazepine produces less weight gain, hair loss, and tremor than valproic acid, and less tremor, urination, and thirst than lithium. The drawbacks of carbamazepine include increased sedation and sense of feeling "drugged." These are all dose-related side effects and can be minimized by decreasing the dose.

Carbamazepine also has a slightly higher incidence of serious side effects and the potential to be fatal in overdose.

Common, Annoying, but not Medically Dangerous Side Effect

Sedation is common, as is some clumsiness and even a sense of confusion. These side effects are dose related and tend to get better within a few days if the person keeps taking the medication.

Nausea is common when the medication is first started but tends to get better or disappear within a week or so.

Medically Dangerous Side Effects

Carbamazepine can interfere with the production of white blood cells. Carbamazepine commonly causes a slight decrease in the white cell count (leukopenia). This usually develops over time, and the white count rarely drops to a dangerous level.

On very rare occasions the person entirely stops making all white blood cells (agranulocytosis). This is reversible if diagnosed in time but fatal if allowed to continue. This is why the white blood cell count is monitored, especially when the medication is started. In addition to the regular blood tests, people starting carbamazepine should be told to get an immediate emergency WBC if they develop a temperature, sore throat, or come down with symptoms that are flu-like. In most cases the white count is normal, but these symptoms of common infections could also be an early sign that the person has stopped making white blood cells, and early detection can literally be life-saving.

Any person taking carbamazepine who gets an infection, fever, sore throat, or mouth sores should immediately get a CBC (complete blood count).

- *Stephens–Johnson Syndrome.* Rashes are relatively common and usually is not a serious concern. Generally the medication does not need to be stopped if a mild rash develops, as long as there is no associated fever, bleeding, or peeling blisters (exfoliative rash). On rare occasions what appears to be a rash can progress to Stevens–Johnson syndrome, a potentially fatal skin reaction. This is significantly more common in people with ancestry from Asia, including South Asian Indians. This is much more common with a particular genetic pattern (HLA-B*1502 gene variant), which can be identified by a simple blood test. This is why anyone with an Asian background should have a test for this genetic pattern before starting carbamazepine. In addition, anyone taking carbamazepine should see a physician immediately if he or she develops a rash that includes mucous membranes, or that includes fever or swollen lymph glands, especially in the first few months of starting the medication.
- *Temporary increases in liver enzymes are common.* Generally liver function tests should be monitored, but the medi-

cation does not need to be stopped unless they are two or three times the normal values. Liver problems are a very rare but potentially dangerous side effect. People taking carbamazepine should be alert to any symptoms of hepatitis, including abdominal tenderness under the right ribs or yellowish skin or eyes.

- *Low sodium (hyponatremia) can occur.* Anyone on carbamazepine who starts feeling very tired or confused should have a serum sodium blood test. Again, this is rare but can become dangerous if the sodium gets too low, and in extreme cases can lead to seizure.

Drug–Drug Interactions

Carbamazepine induces many liver enzymes. This means that over a few weeks it gets the liver increase the ability to deactivate both carbamazepine and other medications. This can lower the blood level of these other medications. *As a result, carbamazepine can interfere with the effectiveness of many oral contraceptives.* Serum levels of many antipsychotics, such as haloperidol, are decreased when carbamazepine is started. It also lowers lamotrigine levels, and the lamotrigine dose is generally doubled when given along with carbamazepine.

Erythromycin, cimetidine, and SSRI antidepressants can all increase the serum level of carbamazepine.

Carbamazepine should not be used in combination with clozapine. There is a concern that the combination may increase the risk of agranulocytosis.

OXCARBAZEPINE (TRILEPTAL)

Oxycarbazepine is one of the metabolites, or breakdown products, of carbamazepine, which has two major metabolic pathways. When carbamazepine is broken apart in the body, one of these pathways leads to pieces or metabolites that are responsible for much of the sedation, confusion, effects on liver and white blood cells caused by carbamazepine. The other pathway of the breakdown leads to oxcarbazepine. The breakdown products from oxcarbazepine are all inactive. The hope is that oxcarbazepine has all of the effectiveness of the original carbamazepine but with fewer side effects. It is clear that oxcarbazepine has fewer side effects than carbamazepine, but there is ongoing debate about whether it is as effective. Although oxcarbazepine is being used more widely as a mood stabilizer, at this moment there is little research clearly showing that it is effective.

If I want to prescribe the medication most likely to be effective, I will typically recommend carbamazepine over oxcarbazepine. If I am most concerned about a medication that will be well tolerated with few side effects, and if the client has the time to try a medication that may be less effective, then oxcarbazepine may be a reasonable choice.

Indications for Use

The primary use of oxcarbazepine in psychiatry is for bipolar disorder and other cyclical mood disorders.

Specifics of Use

There is little information about the best dose of oxcarbazepine. Typically one starts with 300 mg tablets twice a day and then raises the dose as needed until the person's mood is stabler or side effects become a problem. The current maximum dose is 2400 mg/day. Blood levels do not seem very helpful.

Side Effects

Oxcarbazepine has far fewer side effects than carbamazepine. It seems to cause much less sedation and confusion than does carbamazepine. It can induce liver enzymes and lower the blood levels of other medications, including birth control pills, but this effect is much less than that of carbamazepine and is not usually a clinical problem. Oxcarbazepine is much less likely to cause problems with either liver function or white blood cells. Is has been associated with hyponatremia (decreased in serum sodium levels), so serum sodium should be measured every 6 months or so, and a serum sodium level should be ordered between times if the person becomes confused or starts feeling particularly tired.

LAMOTRIGINE (LAMICTAL)

Lamotrigine is an effective anticonvulsant. It is also useful in the treatment of bipolar depression. It is somewhat effective in decreasing the risk of bipolar mania, but it does not seem as effective for this as are other mood stabilizers. It does not seem particularly effective in the treatment of unipolar depression.

Indications for Use

Lamotrigine is currently the treatment of choice for bipolar depression: the depressive side of the bipolar swing. The other mood stabilizers, such as valproic acid or lithium, are very helpful in the manic side of the mood swing, but provide little to no help in treating the depression. Lamotrigine has some effect on the manic side, but it is less effective for mania than valproic acid or lithium.

Bipolar depression is often difficult to treat. Antidepressants are typically less effective with bipolar depression than they are with unipolar depression, and all antidepressants increase the risk of precipitating another manic episode. People with bipolar disorder spend more of their life depressed than manic, and lamotrigine is the first effective treatment for this condition. Although the research has focused on bipolar depression, lamotrigine also seems to be effective for the depressive side of rapid cycling bipolar disorder.

Lamotrigine can be safely combined with the other mood stabilizers for better control of both the "up" and the "down," although dose adjustments must be made to compensate for drug–drug interactions when used with either carbamazepine or valproic acid.

Specifics of Use

It is very important to start lamotrigine at a very low dose and increase very slowly. The biggest risk is Stevens–Johnson syndrome. This often, but not always, begins with a rash, and then proceeds to a very serious rash that can be very dangerous. Stevens–Johnson syndrome is much more likely to develop in the first few months after lamotrigine is started, and it is uncommon after 6 months of continuous medication use. Rashes are common, and most rashes are not the beginning of Stevens–Johnson syndrome and not necessarily dangerous. On the other hand, any rash that begins while starting lamotrigine must be taken seriously. This does not mean that lamotrigine needs to be discontinued after every rash. Rashes are more likely to be dangerous if they involve larger areas of the chest or face, or if they involve the palmer surface of the hands or feet. Any fever with swelling of lymph glands should be taken seriously, and if the rash is accompanied by a fever and swollen lymph glands it should be taken very seriously. This risk of Stevens–Johnson syndrome seems related to how fast the medication is started. If the medication is started at full dose, up to 10% of people starting lamotrigine will develop a potentially dangerous rash. If the medication is stopped, the rash usually goes away without problems. There is also a risk if a person has a gap of 3 or more days off the medication, and then restarts it too rapidly.

Unfortunately, this means that it takes a long time, more than 5 weeks, for a person to get on an effective dose of this medication. Lamotrigine is generally started at 25 mg/day for 2 weeks, then increased to 50 mg/day for another 2 weeks, then increased to 100 mg/day for another week, before increasing it to the normal target dose of 200 mg/day. Then there is yet a further delay once the person is taking this full dose to see if the medication will work. If the person is off lamotrigine for more than 3 days, then this needs to be restarted. There are very convenient starter packs that lay out how much lamotrigine a person should take during the first 4 weeks. A typical dose is 100–200 mg/day for people on lamotrigine alone. Because of enzyme induction, a higher dose is usually needed if lamotrigine is taken along with carbamazepine. Because of enzyme competition, a lower dose is used if taken with valproic acid. There is a specific starter pack designed for people already on an inducer such as carbamazepine, and one for someone on an inhibitor such as valproic acid.

Side Effects

Lamotrigine is usually very well tolerated. Dizziness or double vision are reported, but rarely. Headache is sometimes noted but seems to go away over a few days if the medication is continued. Lamotrigine does not typically cause weight gain or sedation, both problems with some of the other anticonvulsants.

GABAPENTIN (NEURONTIN)

Gabapentin is an effective anticonvulsant. It is used primarily to treat anxiety disorders that have not responded to other interventions, and neurogenic pain.

Indications for Use

Gabapentin is another anticonvulsant that seems to be helpful in a number of psychiatric conditions. At one time there was hope that gabapentin would be an effective mood stabilizer, but the research data are clear that is does not work, at least for most people with classic bipolar disorder. There are anecdotal reports that it may help to stabilize mood in some people with ultra-rapid-cycling disorder (mood shifts every few days or weeks) or mood lability. Unfortunately, there is little research support for this claim.

Gabapentin is useful in anxiety disorders, especially social phobia, and it is helpful for neurogenic pain (that is, pain caused by damaged nerves rather than pain from an arthritic joint or a broken bone). A very common cause of neuropathic pain is diabetic neuropathy, damage to the small nerves from the diabetes. It is also used in the treatment of headaches, and there are some data supporting its use in fibromyalgia, although it is not FDA approved for this use.

Specifics of Use

Gabapentin is used over a wide dose range, from 100 mg twice a day to 1200 mg four times a day. Blood tests do not help identify the best dose. Generally I start gabapentin at 300 mg once or twice a day and then increase every few days until it seems to work. For people who are very sensitive to medication side effects or who are elderly, it can be started at a much lower dose, 100 mg twice a day, to see if it can help with fewer side effects. It is generally taken two or three times a day because of its short half-life.

Side Effects

Gabapentin seems generally well tolerated and safe (even in overdose). Side effects tend to be dose related. It can cause sedation, tiredness, or dizziness in some people, but these are relatively rare. It can cause weight gain, but this is less common and less severe than with some of the other mood stabilizers. It has few drug–drug interactions.

PREGABALIN (LYRICA)

Pregabalin has a similar mode of action to gabapentin, with similar side effects. It is a newer medication, which means that it is expensive and not available as an inexpensive generic, as is gabapentin. It may have fewer side effects than gabapentin for some people, perhaps including less weight gain and less sedation, but there are no good head-to-head studies directly comparing one to another.

Indications for Use

Pregabalin is primarily used as an anticonvulsant, but it is approved for neuropathic pain and fibromyalgia. There are good data indicating that it helps with both the pain and the sleep disruption caused by fibromyalgia. It is similar enough to gabapentin that it is probably effective for some anxiety disorders, although there is not much research support for this application. There are no data indicating that pregabalin is an effective mood stabilizer, and it is not indicated for mood disorders.

Specifics of Use

Pregabalin can be started at a full dose, but the side effects are often less if it is started low and increased over time. Both its effectiveness and its side effects tend to be dose related. A higher does may work better, but is likely to also cause more problems. When used for seizures, the common dose range is 300–600 mg/day. When used for pain, many people experience a significant effect at a much lower dose: 25–100 mg/day is often enough to make a significant difference in the pain of fibromyalgia, and if it is not working at this dose and there are no big problems from side effects. it can then be increased.

Side Effects

Both efficacy and side effects are dose related. The most common side effects are dizziness and tiredness. Weight gain, blurred vision, dry mouth, and constipation are also reported.

TOPIRAMATE (TOPAMAX)

Topirimate is another anticonvulsant that was initially turned to for its perceived mood stabilizing properties. It is not an effective mood stabilizer, however, it may be effective in decreasing impulsive behavior and in reducing headaches and other pain. It also tends to cause weight loss, and is in fact sometimes used expressly for this purpose.

Indications for Use

Topiramate does not appear to be very effective as a mood stabilizer. At one point it appeared that its use in psychiatry was very limited. More recently there has been a suggestion that topiramate may help people control certain kinds of impulsive behavior. There are data showing that it can help some women who chronically cut themselves when upset, and some men with alcohol dependence who impulsively return to drinking.

It is an effective anticonvulsant and is commonly used for control of headaches. Topiramate is one of the very few medications that cause weight loss, and people regularly ask for it for that purpose. It can reverse some of the weight gain caused by other medications, including the weight gain caused by olanzapine and clozapine. Unfortunately, the weight loss is usually modest and may not be sustained over time.

Specifics of Use

It is important to be clear about the target for the topiramate. Is the goal headache relief, decreased chronic cutting or drinking episodes, or weight loss? Topiramate is usually started at 25 mg/day. Some people seem to respond to this low dose, whereas others may need up to 200 mg/day or even more. The side effects are directly related to both dose and how rapidly the dose has been increased.

Side Effects

Many people have significant problems tolerating topiramate. It can cause thinking difficulties in some people, specifically problems finding the right word in the midst of conversation, and problems with memory. I have heard topiramate referred to as "the stupid pill," and several patients have called it "dopamax" instead of Topamax.

Topiramate has been associated with the development of kidney stones and several cases of glaucoma have been reported in people taking topiramate. While this is rare, if it occurs it can cause blindness if not treated rapidly. People taking topiramate should call a physician immediately if eye pain or a change in vision is experienced. It appears that glaucoma is more of a risk in the first month or two after starting the medication, and the risk decreases thereafter.

TIAGABINE (GABITRIL)

Tiagabine is a new anticonvulsant that has been proposed as a mood stabilizer. There is very limited research support for this claim, but tiagabine might be worth trying in an informed person who has already tried all of the more conventional approaches to dealing with mood instability. On the other hand, a number of other anticonvulsants similar to tiagabine were heavily touted as mood stabilizers and then found to be ineffective for this purpose when more data were collected.

There are limited data on the use of tiagabine as a mood stabilizer, but those data that do exist suggest that when it is used as a mood stabilizer it requires a lower dose than when used to control seizures. Most case reports start the medication at 4 mg/day and increase, if necessary, to 8 or 12 mg/day. This is in contrast to the dose range of 16–56 mg/day typically used to control seizures.

Tiagabine appears relatively safe and well tolerated. It has only been used as a mood stabilizer in combination with other medications, so it is a bit difficult to interpret side effects. The most common side effects were dizziness, tiredness, and confusion. Very occasionally, people taking tiagabine for seizures report an increase in depression. All reports of side effects appear rare.

VERAPAMIL

There is a suggestion that calcium channel blockers such as verapamil, which are usually used for treatment of high blood pressure and some heart problems, may also be useful as mood stabilizers. The research support for this is scanty, and there is no suggestion that calcium channel blockers are more effective than the more standard mood stabilizers for most people. On the other hand, if someone has not done well on some of the other mood stabilizers, verapamil may be worth trying. It may also be worth considering the use of verapamil if the person has high blood pressure or some other medical condition that could potentially be treated at the same time by the same medication.

Side Effects

Verapamil is generally well tolerated with relatively few side effects. Most common side effects are dizziness, headache, and nausea. On rare occasions it can cause dangerous arrhythmias (irregular heart rhythm) or liver problems. Loss of energy is sometime reported at higher doses.

Table 6.1 summarizes the salient characteristics and side effects of commonly used mood stabilizers.

TABLE 6.1. Overview of *Common Mood Stabilizers*

	USUAL DOSE (MG/DAY)	SERUM LEVEL	SIDE EFFECTS
Lithium	600–1800	0.6–1.2 mEq/l	Tremor, diarrhea, weight gain, kidney problems, cognitive slowing, thyroid problems
Valproic acid	750–3500	50–120 µg/l	Upset stomach, weight gain, sedation, tremor, hair loss, liver and pancreas problems
Carbamazepine	400–1600	4–12 µg/l	Drowsiness, confusion, dizziness, drop in white blood cells, liver problems
Gabapentin	900–2400	N/A	Tiredness, dizziness
Topiramate	200–400	N/A	Word-finding problems, decreased concentration, kidney stones, glaucoma
Lamotrigine	200–400	N/A	Skin rash, nausea

7

Medications Useful for Anxiety Disorders and Sleep Problems

Until fairly recently, there was not much difference between medications that decreased anxiety (anxiolytics) and those that promoted sleep (hypnotics). Lorazepam (Ativan) and diazepam (Valium) are both benzodiazepines, both are FDA approved as antianxiety medications, and both are also very effective medications to help people get to sleep. Temazepam (Restoril) and flurazepam (Dalmane) are also benzodiazepines; they have the same mechanism of action as lorazepam and diazepam, but both are FDA approved as sleeping medications rather than as antianxiety medications. Many of the medications that have antianxiety properties also have sedative properties. A person can take a small amount of lorazepam during the day to help with anxiety, and a somewhat larger amount before bed to help with sleep.

In the not-so-distant past, there was also not that much difference in the treatment of different kinds of anxiety. It did not matter much if a person had panic disorder or OCD or PTSD; if the person were anxious, he or she would be given diazepam or another similar benzodiazepine. Psychotherapy was similarly nonspecific and pretty much the same across the entire range of anxiety disorders. Treatment is now much more specific, and by understanding the differences it can be much more effective. Just as specific cognitive and behavioral psychotherapy can effectively target specific kinds of anxiety, medications are also targeted with greater precision.

There are now a number of medications that have antianxiety effects but are not sedative (do not induce sleep), and medications that can help sleep but have little to no antianxiety effect. There are also medications that can be useful for some of the symptoms associated with PTSD, and other medications that are specifically useful for performance anxiety. Some of the most effective medications for the treatment of anxiety disorders are antidepressants. As the basic science of sleep and anxiety continues to evolve, more medications will be developed that have very specific desired effects and fewer unwanted side effects.

MEDICATIONS USED PRIMARILY FOR ANXIETY BUT ALSO USED TO PROMOTE SLEEP

All of the benzodiazepines are effective for both promoting sleep and decreasing anxiety. They are more effective at treating panic and generalized anxiety, and less effective in treating OCD. In addition to their anti-anxiety effect, they can also be used to decrease agitation, treat withdrawal from alcohol and other sedative-hypnotic drugs, and to counteract some of the motor restlessness caused by some antipsychotic medications. They are often used outside the realm of psychiatry, to reduce muscle spasms.

Benzodiazepines

Benzodiazepines have both antianxiety and sleep-inducing properties. This drug class includes diazepam (Valium), chlordiazepoxide (Librium), clonazepam (Klonopin), alprazolam (Xanax), flurazepam (Dalmane), and many others. Benzodiazepines are relatively safe medications that are rarely lethal in an overdose, *except when combined with alcohol.*

Benzodiazepines work by binding to a receptor that increases the ability of GABA to inhibit nerve firing. GABA is the primary inhibitory neurotransmitter in the brain. Benzodiazepines do not directly inhibit brain activity; they indirectly inhibit this activity through the GABA system. If there is no GABA at the receptor, a benzodiazepine has very little effect on the neuron. If GABA is present, then the benzodiazepine will amplify the impact of GABA. Because of this indirect effect, an overdose of a benzodiazepine is much safer than an overdose of a medication that directly inhibits brain activity, such as secobarbital (Seconal).

GABA receptors are large, complicated structures. Benzodiazepines can bind to a number of different sites within these GABA receptors. When a benzodiazepine attaches to a GABA receptor, it changes the shape of the receptor to make it more receptive to the activity of GABA. GABA receptors are located on neurons that decrease anxiety, promote sleep onset, decrease muscle spasms, and have an anticonvulsant property. This means that a benzodiazepine that nonspecifically attaches to sites on different kinds of GABA receptors will decrease anxiety, but it will also make the person tired. Whether this is a therapeutic effect or a side effect depends on whether this effect is desired or perceived as a problem.

Benzodiazepines, barbiturates, and many medications used as sleeping pills or antianxiety medications can be addicting and are subject to abuse. It is important to put this risk of abuse into perspective. All of the antianxiety medications now in widespread use are much less addicting and much less dangerous than alcohol. Like alcohol, most people can use these medications safely with little risk, even over long periods of time, but some people do get into abuse patterns and become dependent.

Benzodiazepines are all at least partially cross-tolerant with each other and with alcohol (an addicted individual can replace one medication with another). Withdrawal from these sedative medications is much more medically dangerous than opiate withdrawal. Abruptly stopping the use of medications in someone who is addicted to alcohol, barbiturates, or diazepam (Valium) can result in life-threatening convulsions. If addiction to any of these medications is a possibility, medication for a gradual detoxification should be prescribed. At times, hospital admission may be necessary to control drug use during the withdrawal period.

Differences among Benzodiazepines

Benzodiazepines all work the same way and seem to bind to pretty much the same receptors. Alprazolam (Xanax) seems to be more subject to abuse than other benzodiazepines. Clonazepam

(Klonopin) is a long-acting, sedating benzodiazepine that is sometimes used as an anticonvulsant. The major differences between them have to do with how long they take to get into the brain and start working, and how long their effects last (measured as half-life, or the time it takes for the body to eliminate 50% of the medication). A number of factors can affect the speed of onset and duration. For example, most medications are absorbed faster on an empty stomach than following a big meal. After a medication is absorbed from the stomach and into the blood, how fast it gets into the brain is influenced by how "fat soluble" the medication is. The brain is protected from the blood by a "blood–brain barrier" that is made up of very modified fat cells. A medication that is very fat soluble, such as diazepam (Valium), will get from the blood into the brain much faster than a medication that is less fat soluble such as chlordiazepoxide (Librium). Duration of action for most medications depends on how long it takes for the liver to break them down into inactive pieces or how long it takes the kidneys to excrete than in the urine.

Some medications have a further complication. For example, diazepam has a different duration of action depending on whether it is used occasionally or daily. For the occasional user, diazepam's duration is limited by redistribution. Diazepam rapidly leaves active sites on nerve cells and, since it is very fat soluble, is absorbed by fat cells all over the body. After chronic use, these fat cells become saturated, and duration is limited by the speed with which the medication is broken down by the liver, a much longer process. In the occasional user, diazepam is a short-acting medication, but for the chronic user it is a long-acting medication. Oxazepam (Serax) has a shorter duration of action (half-life) than most of the others. Flurazepam (Dalmane) has a rapid onset and a very long half-life, so, although it is sold as a sleeping pill, it has significant anxiolytic (antianxiety) action for the next day or 2. Both diazepam and chlordiazepoxide have moderately long half-lives. The effective half-lives of many medications such as diazepam are extended by the presence of active metabolites. That is, the medication is broken down into other chemicals that continue to have sedative and antianxiety effects.

A benzodiazepine that acts rapidly will be felt by the person as "doing something," whereas a slower-onset medication is often perceived to be less effective because the person does not feel a "kick." On the other hand, rapid-onset sedative hypnotics tend to be more addicting than similar medications with a slower onset of action. When a long-acting medication such as flurazepam is given to help with sleep, it can cause a significant hangover the next day, and when given several nights in a row, it can build up in the person and cause tiredness or confusion. A hangover can be avoided by using a very short-acting medication such as triazolam (Halcion). However, when used as a sleeping pill, a short-acting medication can cause the person to wake up partway through the night with rebound insomnia, as the brain reacts to the rapid decrease in medication level. Table 7.1 provides an overview of commonly prescribed benzodiazepines.

TABLE 7.1. *Profiles of Common Benzodiazepines*

	HALF-LIFE (HOURS)	DOSE RANGE (MG)	SPEED OF ONSET	ADDICTION POTENTIAL
alprazolam (Xanax)	9–20	0.5–4	+ + +	Higher
chlordiaz-epoxide (Librium)	28–100	15–100	+ +	Lower
clonazepam (Klonopin)	19–60	1.5–4	+ +	Moderate
diazepam (Valium)	30–200	2–40	+ + + +	Higher
lorazepam (Ativan)	8–24	1–4	+ +	Moderate
oxazepam (Serax)	3–25	30–60	+	Lower

Note: speed of onset is strongly influenced by many factors. All of these medications will be absorbed more quickly on an empty stomach. Most act more quickly on a person with less regular benzodiazepam or alcohol use. Diazepam is likely to have an initial effect within 30 minutes of ingestion on an empty stomach. Chlordiazepoxide will typically take well over an hour to have significant pharmacological effect.

Indications for Use

There are six major categories of benzodiazepine application:
1. Anxiety
    General anxiety
    Panic
    Anticipatory anxiety associated with panic
    Anxiety secondary to stress
2. Sleep
3. Side effects of other medications
4. Agitation
5. Alcohol and other sedative/hypnotic withdrawal
6. Muscle spasms

Benzodiazepines are most commonly used to decrease anxiety, for which they are very effective. They decrease anxiety whether it is caused by stress, generalized anxiety disorder, or anticipatory anxiety connected to panic disorder. They are easily used and well tolerated. People tend to like taking a benzodiazepine. One of the concerns is that some people want to use a benzodiazepine to cover over a problem, instead of trying to change something to solve the problem. It is, of course, an issue of personal values what things should be changed, and what things are appropriate to cover over. Just as a bandage can help a cut have time to heal, a benzodiazepine can similarly give a person time and capacity to cope more effectively. Many people with chronic anxiety have a much more comfortable life with the use of these medications. It is important to understand the nature and cause of the person's anxiety and whether the medication is helping the person live more effectively or getting in the way of how he or she is living. It is important for the consumer, the prescriber, and others in the person's support system to discuss these issues and be clear how the medication can help and in what ways it cannot.

Benzodiazepines are generally not very helpful in people with obsessive–compulsive disorder (OCD). They do not tend to decrease the obsessive or compulsive behavior, and for most people do not help very much even with the associated anxiety. Moreover, there is concern that they can actually interfere with the behavioral therapies that are the cornerstone of effective OCD treatment. Some of the antidepressants, especially the SSRIs and clomipramine (Anafranil), can be useful, but benzodiazepines should generally not be used for treatment of OCD.

Panic Disorder
Any of the benzodiazepines will decrease the intensity and frequency of panic attacks. Such attacks typically last only a few minutes, so if a person takes a pill of diazepam at the moment the attack starts, it would not have time to take action before the attack would have ended on its own. For a benzodiazepine to be to effective to prevent or shorten a panic attack, it must be taken before the panic attack occurs—which usually means taking it every day. Benzodiazepines can also help a person cope with the anticipatory anxiety that comes from the fear of having another panic attack. Such anxiety can be very distressing and even disabling.

Whereas some clinicians use benzodiazepines as a first-line medication for panic, I prefer to start with one of the SSRI-type antidepressant medications, which are equally effective and not subject to abuse.

Sleep
All of the benzodiazepines have both antianxiety and sedating properties. Some are marketed and FDA approved as a hypnotic (sleeping pill) whereas others are not, but they will all help someone get to sleep. Of course, it is important to make sure that the person does not have a medical problem such as sleep apnea or COPD (chronic obstructive pulmonary disease) that is the cause of the sleep problem and could be made worse by any sleeping pill. It is also important to understand the cause of the sleep disruption, especially if it is a chronic problem. A problem of circadian rhythms, whereby the person's body wants to sleep at the wrong time of day, can be better handled by different medications or by trying to adjust timing of the

person's sleep cycle. Some people use sleep as a way to avoid boredom, and they complain of not being able to sleep when they are actually sleeping more than 9 hours a night. Heavy smokers may wake up during the night as their body reacts to the effects of nicotine withdrawal. People often use alcohol as a way of trying to get to sleep, but it actually disrupts the sleep cycle throughout the night. Keeping a sleep diary for a while can be very helpful in understanding the pattern of the sleep disruption.

Sleep disruption can be very distressing. Someone who is depressed and not sleeping will feel much better, and be better able to cope with the depression, if he or she is helped to sleep while waiting for an antidepressant to take effect. Not sleeping can also precipitate a manic episode in someone who has a bipolar illness, and using a medication to get back into a regular sleep pattern can be an important part of preventing that episode.

Side Effects of Other Medications

Benzodiazepines such as clonazepam or lorazepam can decrease the agitation that can be the temporary side effect of some of the more activating antipsychotic medications such as ziprasidone (Geodon) or aripiprazole (Abilify). Some antidepressants, including the SSRIs and SNRIs, can also induce some early agitation and sleep disruption that usually pass within a few days but can be uncomfortable and are easily treated with short-term use of a benzodiazepine. Even when they do not make anxiety or sleep worse, all of the antidepressants take some time to work. Again, the short-term use of a benzodiazepine to decrease anxiety and stabilize sleep can lead to a faster onset of action and help the person become more comfortable more rapidly.

Akathisia is a particularly uncomfortable side effect that is most commonly caused by antipsychotic medication. On rare occasions akathisia is also associated with antidepressant medications. It is a motor restlessness that makes the person feel as if he or she has to keep moving, walking, or rocking even when tired. It is so uncomfortable that it often causes the person to discontinue the medication that seems to be causing it. The initial treatment for akathisia is to try to decrease the dose of the medication causing it, and to decrease the use of caffeine or other medications or drugs that might be making it worse. If this does not work, a number of medications can be tried. A beta-blocker such as propranolol (Inderal) or an anticholinergic medication such as benztropine (Cogentin) will often work, but benzodiazepines also work and are usually well tolerated.

Agitation
Benzodiazepines are effective ways to help decrease agitation, whether the cause of that agitation is from a psychosis or from an upsetting experience. Benzodiazepines should be used with caution, however, for in agitation associated with dementia or delirium these medications can also cause disinhibition. Like alcohol, some people end up doing things while taking a benzodiazepine that they would not otherwise do.

Alcohol and Other Sedative/Hypnotic Withdrawal
As noted, all benzodiazepines are cross-tolerant with each other and with alcohol. Alcohol withdrawal for someone who is seriously dependent on either alcohol or any of the benzodiazepines can be both uncomfortable and dangerous. In extreme cases, a person can develop life-threatening seizures from this withdrawal. It is possible to slowly and safely taper the person's use of alcohol or the drug on which he or she is dependent, but doing so is cumbersome. It is more common and safer to substitute any of the benzodiazepines for the alcohol, and then taper off that medication in a controlled way. The important issue is to complete the taper so that the person is not now dependent on the benzodiazepine that was used for the taper.

Muscle Spasms
There are a number of nonpsychiatric uses for the benzodiazepines, one of which is to decrease muscle spasms. This is a common use after a back injury or in the ongoing treatment of multiple sclerosis or cerebral palsy.

Specifics of Use

As with all medications, benzodiazepines should not be used without a reason and should not be continued without a reason for continuation.

Diazepam (Valium)

As an antianxiety medication, diazepam is commonly prescribed in 5 or 10 mg tablets up to 40 mg/day. It is absorbed much faster by mouth than by intramuscular injection. It can be used intravenously to stop a seizure. Because it is very fat soluble, it gets into the brain rapidly, which means that a person "feels" it more than some of the others. As a result, it is somewhat more abusable than some of the others. It may have more potential to decrease muscle spasms than other benzodiazepines and is the one commonly prescribed for this purpose.

Chlordiazepoxide (Librium)

Chlordiazepoxide is prescribed in doses of 10–25 mg up to 100 mg/day. It is one of the oldest medications in this class. For unclear reasons it has dropped out of favor. It has a slow onset time and a long half-life. This means that it does not "hit" as rapidly when first taken, and it also has a lower abuse potential.

Lorazepam (Ativan)

Lorazepam has an intermediate half-life of approximately 14 hours, which is long enough that there is not a fast peak, and short enough that there is little accumulation from day-to-day when it is used over multiple days. Usually given in 0.5–2 mg tablets two or three times a day, it is well tolerated. Like all of the benzodiazepines it has phamacodynamic interactions, which means that when taken with another sedating medication, the effects can add be additive. Lorazepam does not have any significant pharmacokinetic interactions—which means that other medications do not change the serum level of the lorazepam. It is well absorbed both by mouth and by intramuscular injection. It has become a common medication to use in crisis situations, where it can be given give either by mouth or by injection to rapidly decrease agitation.

Clonazepam (Klonopin)
Clonazepam is rapidly absorbed and slowly metabolized with a half-life of 19–60 hours. This means that if taken daily, the serum level is likely to increase over the first 5–10 days of use. This long half-life has the potential advantage of producing a steadier serum level than a shorter-acting medication. It is usually prescribed in 0.5–2 mg tablets once or twice a day, up to 4 mg/day.

Alprazolam (Xanax)
When alprazolam is used as an antianxiety medication, a typical dose range is 1–4 mg/day in divided doses. When it is used as an anti-panic medication, it may be necessary to use a higher dose. Alprazolam has a somewhat higher abuse potential than most benzodiazepines. It seems a bit easier to get "hooked" and a bit harder to get off it. At the same time, it is very well tolerated and most people taking it do not abuse it and do not become dependent. In general, if someone comes to me on alprazolam and is doing well, I will continue it, but I prefer to use other benzodiazepines.

Side Effects
- *All of the benzodiazepines are addictive*, but to put things into perspective, diazepam (Valium) is less addicting and certainly less dangerous than alcohol. The shorter-acting benzodiazepines such as alprazolam (Xanax) are more addicting than the longer-acting medications in the same class. Medications with a "kick" caused by their rapid onset of action, such as diazepam, seem somewhat more subject to abuse than medications with a more gradual onset, such as chlordiazepoxide (Librium). A person who has been taking any of these medications for more than a few days should decrease it slowly rather than stop it abruptly. Serious, at times life-threatening, seizures from abrupt withdrawal have been reported with all of the benzodiazepines, but these are more likely with shorter-acting medications such as alprazolam than longer-acting medications such as clonaze-

pam. A gradual withdrawal is safer and also helps to minimize the inevitable discomfort that accompanies it.

- *All of the benzodiazepines may cause drowsiness* (which usually improves after a few days of use). People should be warned about using machinery or driving cars, especially when getting used to these medications.
- *All of these medications cause an intoxication similar to that of alcohol,* with impaired judgment, decreased coordination, light-headedness, etc. Recent research has suggested that even people well adjusted to small doses of these medications have a small but measurable impairment in their driving ability. A similar slight impairment is caused by a glass of wine or a beer, even though the person is not near the legal limit of intoxication and does not feel at all impaired. These effects wear off quickly; with shorter-acting medications and remain much longer with the longer-acting medications.
- *Benzodiazepines can sometimes unleash otherwise inhibited behavior.* Again, this disinhibition is similar to, but less severe than, the disinhibition that occurs with alcohol intoxication.
- *All of these medications can interfere with memory.* This effect seems to be of most concern with older people who might already have some memory impairment. There are scatted reports of people doing things under the influence of these medications that they cannot remember later. This effect is similar to sleepwalking but can involve more complex behaviors over a longer period of time. Reported behaviors include driving a car or having an extended conversation. At times these behaviors can be dangerous—not intentionally but because of poor judgment during the episode. Shorter-acting benzodiazepines, particularly triazolam (Halcion), have been most commonly associated with this problem.

Use during Pregnancy

It has been suggested that these medications might increase birth defects, although recent reviews have found no evidence of this claim. Nevertheless, when possible as a precaution, benzodiazepines should be avoided by pregnant women, especially during the first 3 months of pregnancy.

MEDICATIONS USEFUL FOR ANXIETY BUT NOT FOR SLEEP

It was once commonly assumed that any medication that decreased anxiety would also increase drowsiness, but it is now known that this is not necessarily true. Buspirone is effective in reducing general anxiety, but it has no effect on sleep and does not reduce panic or other specific anxiety disorders. The beta-blockers, such as propranolol (inderal), decrease performance-related anxiety but not other types of anxiety. D-cycloserine can facilitate behavioral treatment for OCD. It is anticipated that other specific, non-sedating antianxiety medications will be developed in the near future.

Buspirone (BuSpar)

Buspirone works through a different mechanism of action than either the benzodiazepines or other sedative/hypnotics. It partially stimulates (is a partial agonist) of the $5HT_{1A}$ serotonin receptor. It is nonaddictive, not habit forming, and not subject to abuse. It is anxiolytic (anxiety reducing) without being sedating. It does not appear to make people more sensitive to the effects of alcohol or other sedating medications. It is not a muscle relaxant and has no anticonvulsant properties. It is also not useful in helping with alcohol or other drug withdrawal.

Buspirone may be useful in augmenting the effectiveness of antidepressant medications, although the data to support this possibility are very limited. There is also anecdotal suggestion that it could be used to reverse the sexual side effects of SSRI antidepressants, especially in women, but again there is little research support for this use.

Buspirone does appear to have a few idiosyncrasies that may limit its use. Whereas diazepam (Valium) and the other benzodiazepines appear to work almost immediately, buspirone must be used regularly for up to several weeks before it is fully effective. This means it is best used as a regular medication for someone who can tolerate a delay before it begins working, rather than as a medication with rapid effects that can be taken episodically, as with benzodiazepines.

A second issue has to do with its effectiveness. Double-blind research studies have concluded that buspirone is as effective as diazepam when used by anxious subjects who have never previously used diazepam. For some reason, people who have previously had much experience with benzodiazepines often feel that buspirone is less effective. There are at least two possible interpretations of these research findings. One is that the use of benzodiazepines produces long-lasting biological changes in the brain that make buspirone less effective, and the other is that buspirone is not really quite as effective as benzodiazepines, but that it works "well enough" for most people, unless they have experience with something else to compare it to.

Buspirone seems particularly useful for people who are potential drug abusers and for those who do not like or cannot tolerate the sedative side effects of benzodiazepines. This medication is most often used in an attempt to augment the effectiveness of other medications.

Specifics of Use

Buspirone can be started at 10 mg twice a day, and then increased after a few days. It is more likely to be effective at 40–60 mg day then at a lower dose. The FDA upper limit is 60 mg/day, but it seems safe at a higher dose, and some people find a higher dose more effective.

Side Effects

Buspirone is generally well tolerated. It can cause some dizziness, drowsiness, nausea, or headache, but only rarely.

Beta-blockers

Beta-blockers—propranolol (Inderal), atenolol (Tenormin)—are used primarily in performance anxiety, that is, anxiety that is specific to giving a public talk or taking an exam. Beta-blockers may also have a role in treating generalized anxiety when there is a significant somatic component (sweating, racing heart, etc.) to the anxiety. These medications affect the feedback loop between the body and the brain and have little direct effect on the brain itself. They work rapidly, can be used only when symptoms arise, and have few mental side effects such as sedation or cognitive impairment. They are not addicting or abusable and are generally safe, even in an overdose. (See chapter 7 for more details)

D-Cycloserine

D-cycloserine increases the effectiveness of behavioral therapy for OCD. It does not appear effective when this medication is used alone, but only when it is combined with behavioral therapy. In research studies involving d-cycloserine, the behavioral therapy consisted of 10 sessions focused on exposure and response prevention. This finding of the positive effect of d-cycloserine is in contrast to the effects of benzodiazepines, which seem to interfere with the effectiveness of behavioral therapy.

   D-cycloserine is an NMDA receptor agonist. Much more will be heard about NMDA agonists in the next few years. Briefly, the primary activating neurotransmitter in the brain is glutamate. Too much excitatory activity can kill nerve cells, but some activity is necessary for any learning. NMDA receptors are one of the major glutamate receptors, and d-cycloserine (or glycine) is required for glutamate to activate this receptor type. D-cycloserine can potentially be used to enhance certain kinds of learning in very selected situations, and, as noted, there are now good data that this medication is a useful adjunct to behavioral therapy. Specifically, the medication increases the extinction of anxiety that is part of the behavioral therapy paradigm. This work on d-cycloserine is the beginning of new ways to look at brain circuitry and the interaction of medications and therapy. It suggests that there are specific brain pathways that underlie OCD, and that both medication and behavioral therapy can affect that pathway, in different ways. It is important not to oversimplify these very complicated systems, however; there are no data that d-cycloserine improves other kinds of learning, or other kinds of fear.

Antidepressants as Antianxiety Medications

All of the antidepressants, with the exception of bupropion (Wellbutrin), are very effective antianxiety medications. As discussed in Chapter 4, antidepressants are effective antianxiety medications even for people who are not depressed. Besides helping with generalized anxiety, as a group they are also effective with panic. The antidepressants with serotonin activity, including the SSRIs such as fluoxetine (Prozac) and the SNRIs such as venlafaxine (Effexor), are much more effective than the benzodiazepines for symptoms of obsessive–compulsive disorder (OCD). Clomipramine (Anafranil) is an older antidepressant with significant serotonin activity that is at least as effective at the SSRIs for OCD.

Antidepressants can take several weeks to work and may have more side effects than benzodiazepines. On the other hand, they are not addictive and not subject to being abused. These characteristics make them the medication of choice for people with a history of alcohol abuse or other addictive disorder.

Most of the newer antidepressants have relatively little sedative effect, and although they can help stabilize sleep by treating an underlying depression or anxiety disorder, they are not useful as sleeping pills, per se. The more sedating antidepressants can help a person sleep while also helping with depression and anxiety. Mirtazapine (Remeron) is very sedating and therefore particularly useful for sleep, although the weight gain associated with it is sometimes a problem.

MEDICATIONS USEFUL FOR SLEEP BUT NOT ANXIETY

Hypnotics (Sleeping Pills)

It is important to assess the nature of the sleep problem before deciding that the solution is to prescribe a sleeping pill. Many people who complain of insomnia are already sleeping an adequate amount but feel that they "should" be sleeping more. In some cases a person may be sleeping as much as his or her body needs, but he or she is trying to use sleep to fill up time. Other people are concerned that they cannot sleep at night but are taking naps during the day; in these cases the problem is the structure of the sleep cycle rather than a lack of sleep. Other people are depressed, and the insomnia usually improves when the depression is treated. Some people with insomnia have a specific sleep disorder, such as sleep apnea or restless leg syndrome. There are specific treatments for these disorders, and sleeping pills may actually make things worse.

Sleep apnea is of special concern because it is fairly common and can cause significant medical problems as well as depression and daytime sleepiness. Most people with sleep apnea have a pattern of heavy snoring interrupted by periods of not breathing, repeated many times during the night. It is most common in people who are overweight, and the best clues often come from the snoring patterns described by the person's bed partner.

Sleeping pills are frequently necessary in the hospital because of the noise and strangeness of the environment and the general anxiety of the person. Nevertheless, they should not be prescribed automatically, and they should not be used with anyone who is still intoxicated with alcohol or any other depressant. Sleeping pills should be used with caution in older people, who are likely to become confused or disoriented, or, on rare occasions, slip into a terrifying transient organic psychosis. Finally, people with severe respiratory diseases are more apt to develop serious medical complications from the respiratory-depressant side effects of many medications, especially sleeping pills.

Insomnia can be a short-term or a chronic problem. The idea of chronic insomnia requiring ongoing treatment is somewhat new, but is now well accepted by sleep experts. When I prescribe sleeping pills for someone going through a situational disturbance, I rarely give more than five pills at a time. It is sometimes nice to have a sleeping pill in the medicine closet for especially bad nights. Some people do benefit from the use of a sleeping pill on a regular basis, but I am cautious about their long-term use. I want to be clear about the nature of the sleep disorder before starting what may become long-term treatment with a medication that can have side effects and can mask the real problem. Often, the problems caused by sleeping pills are worse than the problems caused by poor sleep.

Commonly used sleeping pills can be divided into five categories: benzodiazepines, which are nonspecific boosters of GABA activity and can help with both sleep and anxiety; specific GABA-A receptor agonists that have much bigger effects on sleep than on anxiety; sedating antidepressants; medications that change the circadian rhythm and signal the brain that it is time for sleep; and over the counter sleeping pills that are either antihistaminic or anticholinergic medications. Of course, a large number of other drugs and medications have sedative properties. Barbiturates such as secobarbital (Seconal) are now rarely used and are much more dangerous and addictive than their more modern replacements. Alcohol is the most common drug used to promote sleep, but while it can help promote sleep onset, it can actually disrupt sleep architecture.

Benzodiazepines Used as Sleeping Pill

As previously discussed, all of the benzodiazepines are both sedating and anxiolytic (antianxiety), and all of them can and are used to promote sleep. Some are specifically marketed as a sleeping pill, such as flurazepam (Dalmane) or temazepam (Restoril). Others, such as lorazepam or diazepam, are marketed and approved for their antianxiety effect. It does not matter—they all work. However, there are important differences in their speed of onset and duration of action.

- *Flurazepam (Dalmane).* The active metabolite of flurazepam has a half-life of 40–250 hours. This means that if someone takes it every night, the effective serum level of the medication keeps increasing for weeks. This problem is worse in older people, who can become confused and appear demented if they take flurazepam nightly to help them sleep, and as a result they end up with a higher and higher serum level. The usual dose is 15 mg before bed.

- *Triazolam (Halcion)* has an extremely fast onset time and a very short half-life of 1.5 hours. It has been associated with more memory problems than the other medications in this same class. It is also associated with more sleepwalking and other complex sleep activities. Finally, its very short onset–offset makes it more subject to abuse than other benzodiazepines. For all of these reasons, I do not prescribe triazolam, even when people have used it successfully in the past.

- *Temazepam (Restoril)* is a relatively short-acting benzodiazepine that is both safe and effective. The short half-life means that the medication does not accumulate from one night to the next, as does flurazepam. The usual dose is 15 mg before bedtime, although increasing to 30 mg is not unusual. It may be a bit more addictive than the more selective medications, such as zolpidem or zaleplon (next section).

Selective GABA-A Agonists

Benzodiazepines bind to a number of sites on the GABA receptor. Selective GABA receptor hypnotics bind selectively to those parts of the GABA receptor that affect sleep, and do not bind to those sites that affect anxiety or seizures. These selective GABA agonists seem less likely to be abused and to produce dependence. In addition to this lower abuse potential, the selective GABA hypnotics may be more likely than the nonselective benzodiazepines to keep working as an effective sleep agent, even if used over a long period of time.

Concern has been raised about reports of taking one of these medications and then driving or performing other complex activities without any recollection. It is behavior somewhat similar to sleepwalking and can theoretically lead to risky or dangerous outcomes. This effect seems to be rare, and it is probably a risk with all of the sleeping agents in this class.

- *Zolpidem (Ambien)* is effective, nonaddicting, and lacking in significant side effects. Tolerance does not seem to develop to zolpidem, and it continues to be effective even when taken nightly for long periods of time. For a healthy adult, 10 mg is a typical dose and 5 mg is a typical geriatric dose. Some people may need up to 20 mg. It is now available as an inexpensive generic medication.

Zolpidem is also available in a controlled-release form, designed so that part of the medication is released immediately and part of it is released slowly over several hours. Called *Ambien CR,* this tablet is only available as a brand name product and is therefore much more expensive than the regular release, generic version of the same medication.

- *Zaleplon (Sonata)* is very similar to zolpidem. It is related to, but different from benzodiazepines and is a highly effective sleeping pill with little antianxiety action. It has an even shorter half-life than zolpidem. This means that if someone takes zolpidem and feels "hung over" the next morning, zaleplon may be a better choice. If someone takes zaleplon and wakes up in the middle of the night, than the slightly longer action of zolpidem may be a better choice. A typical dose is 5–10 mg before bedtime, although 20 mg may be needed for some people.
- *Eszopiclone (Lunesta)* has a slightly longer half-life than the other medications in this group, which means that it may help maintain sleep throughout the night, but is also a bit more likely to lead to some sedation the next morning. A typical dose is 2 or 3 mg before bedtime.

Sedating Antidepressants

A number of antidepressants are very sedating. Many people who are depressed have a significant problem with sleep, so using a medication that both treats the depression and helps with sleep makes a lot of sense. The use of these medications for people who are not depressed is a bit more controversial. There is not much research on the long-term effect of these medications on sleep, and they are not FDA approved for use as sleeping pills, but they are used very frequently for this purpose, and they seem to work well.

• *Trazodone (Desyrel)* is a sedative antidepressant that is commonly used as a safe and effective hypnotic. In fact, it is more commonly used for sleep than as an antidepressant. For sleep, a typical dose is 50–100 mg taken before bedtime. When taken only at night, it is short-acting enough to cause little sedation, typically, the next morning. To be effective as an antidepressant it must be taken at 300–600 mg/day in divided doses several times during the day. It is a very sedating, so when it is used as an antidepressant, sedation is a major side effect.

  The advantages of trazodone are that it is not addicting and not abusable, and it *is* inexpensive, generally well tolerated, and usually works well. It does have some side effects. When used regularly, especially in higher doses, it can cause some weight gain. Like all antidepressants there is a very small risk that it could precipitate a manic episode in someone who is predisposed to becoming manic. The most concerning side effect is specific to males: the very small risk of priapism. In rare cases, trazodone can cause prolonged, painful, and potentially damaging erections that may need surgical intervention and can lead to permanent impotency. Any man taking trazodone should be warned about this very rare side effect, and if he experiences unusually prolonged erections, the medication should be stopped.

• *Mirtazapine (Remeron)* is an effective antidepressant that is very sedating. (See Chapter 4 on antidepressants for a more complete discussion.) It is a very good choice when trying to decide which antidepressant to use in someone who is depressed or anxious. It is sometimes used solely for its hypnotic properties, but it has significant weight gain as a side effect, and in general there are safer alternatives if promoting sleep is the only concern.

• *Amitriptyline (Elavil) and doxepin (Sinequan)* are older tricyclic antidepressant medications. (See Chapter 4 on antidepressants for a more complete discussion.) A number of the tricyclic antidepressants are sedating and can be used for sleep. They work, are not addictive, and are not subject to abuse. They also have significant side effects, and are dangerous if taken in an overdose. Although the use of sedating tricyclic antidepressants as sleeping aids is not uncommon, I do not recommend them in the absence of depression or pain or some other reason that would support their use.

Melatonin and Medications that Work on Melatonin Receptors

Melatonin

Melatonin is one of the neurotransmitters that tells the brain that it is time to go to sleep. It is released by the pineal gland in the brain in response to darkness, and is shut off in response to light. For most people, natural melatonin levels drop in the evening and rise in the morning before awakening. People with disruptions in their sleep–wake cycle often have a disruption in when melatonin is released. Ensuring the presence of light in the morning before awakening and going to sleep in a dark room can restore this cycle of melatonin release.

Melatonin has been available as a health food for some time. It is effective in helping people nudge their circadian rhythms to fit their lifestyle. For example, melatonin is useful for people with work schedules that require that they modify their normal bedtime, or people who travel to different time zones and suffer jet lag that disrupts their normal sleep pattern. Melatonin is generally considered both safe and effective, but there are some problems with its use as a sleeping aid. The doses obtained in the over-the-counter preparations are not always reliable, and there is considerable debate about the best dose. There is also concern that melatonin may have some tendency to make depression or mood lability worse.

Ramelteon (Rozerem)

Natural melatonin affects three different melatonin receptors. Ramelteon is a prescription medication that stimulates two of these melatonin receptors, M1 and M2, and has little activity on the M3 receptor. The normal dose is 8 mg, taken approximately 30 minutes before going to bed. Like melatonin, it generally works better if taken for several days. It is not absorbed if taken with, or shortly after, a high-fat meal. It has no addiction or abuse potential and seems a safe and effective way to promote sleep. Since it has a very different mechanism of action than other sleeping pills, it may work better for some people than for others.

There is some concern that, like melatonin, ramelteon can make depression worse. This does not seem to be a common problem and, in general, the medication seems to have few side effects for most people. The major issue is whether it is effective.

Antihistamines

Antihistamines, not surprisingly, block histamines. Blocking histamine receptors causes sedation, and stimulating histamine receptors promotes wakefulness. The sedating effect of antihistamines is usually considered a side effect, but it can be used to promote sleep, and many of the over-the-counter sleeping aids and nighttime cold medications that are designed to help induce sleep contain antihistamines.

Diphenhydramine (Benadryl) is the most commonly used sedating antihistamine. The biggest problem with it, and the other sedating antihistamines, is its anticholinergic side effects (blocks the action of acetylcholine). These include dry mouth, constipation, and blurred vision. More importantly, anticholinergic medications such as diphenhydramine can also cause confusion, especially in the elderly or in people who are already taking other anticholinergic medications (including many of the antidepressants or antipsychotic medications). Diphenhydramine has already been mentioned as a treatment for muscular side effects from antipsychotic medications. The recommended dose is 50–100 mg before bedtime, with instructions that the person may repeat that dose in one hour.

Table 7.1 provides a summary of commonly prescribed sleeping pills.

TABLE 7.1. *Profiles of Common Sleeping Pills*

	DOSE RANGE (MG)	HALF-LIFE (HR.)
Benzodiazepine Sleeping Pills		
Estazolam (Prosom)	1–2	8–24
Flurazepam (Dalmane)	15–30	48–120
Quazepam (Doral)	7.5–15	48–120
Temazepam (Restoril)	7.5–30	8–20
Triazolam (Halcion)	0.125–0.25	2–4
Selective GABAA Agonist (nonbenzodiazepine) Sleeping Pills		
Eszopiclone (Lunesta)	1–3	5–7
Zaleplon (Sonata)	5–10	1
Zolpidem (Ambien)(a)	5–10	1.5–2.4
Zolpidem ER (Ambien CR)	6.25–12.5	2.8–2.9
Selective Melatonin Receptor Agonist		
Ramelteon (Rozerem)	8	1–2.6
Sedating Antidepressants(b)		
Trazodone (Desyrel)	50–100	
Mirtazapine (Remeron)	15–30	
Doxepin Sinequan)	50–150	

a. Available as inexpensive generic
b. Not FDA approved as hypnotic but often used as such

8

Miscellaneous Medications

A few medications are important to include in this book, but they do not neatly fit into one of the four categories. These are all somewhat "special purpose" medications that are a bit outside of the basic treatment of mental illness. I discuss six categories of miscellaneous medications:

- Medications for EPS, motor side effects of antipsychotic medications
- Beta-blockers (e.g., propranolol [Inderal] for performance anxiety, tremor, and akathisia)
- Medications for PTSD
- Medications for ADHD
- Medications for Alzheimer's disease
- Medications to treat alcohol dependence and substance abuse

MEDICATIONS FOR THE MOTOR SIDE EFFECTS OF ANTIPSYCHOTIC MEDICATIONS

Some of the medications commonly used for Parkinson's disease are also useful in treating the Parkinson-like (*parkinsonian*, to refer to these medication side effects), muscle-related side effects of the antipsychotic medications. Parkinson's disease is caused by the loss of dopamine-containing cells in that part of the brain that controls involuntary muscle coordination. Antipsychotic medications do not kill off these cells, but they do block the effect of dopamine on receptors, which functionally causes similar symptoms. The second-generation or atypical antipsychotic medications, since they are much more selective about where in the brain they decrease dopamine, are much less likely to cause parkinsonian side effects. As a result, the need for anticholinergic medication is much less with the second-generation medications than it is with the older medications. Some people do get parkinsonian or motor side effects even with the atypical antipsychotics, especially when the dose is raised. In addition, first-generation antipsychotic medications continue to be used. Some data suggest that the outcome differences between the first- and second-generation medications may not be as clear as was once thought, and many people with schizophrenia appear to do as well on the older medications as they do on the newer ones; in fact, some people even do better with the older medications.

As was already discussed, the extrapyramidal muscle-related side effects include dystonias (muscle spasms), tremors, akathisia (motor restlessness), and akinesia (decreased spontaneity of movements and thought). All of these are connected to a decrease in the availability of dopamine. Tardive dyskinesia, the potentially permanent movement that are a long-term risk with the use of any antipsychotic medication, is thought to be the result of a different mechanism and is generally not helped by antiparkinsonian medications.

Anticholinergics

Many of the antiparkinsonian medications used in psychiatry are anticholinergic; that is, they block acetylcholine receptors throughout the body (cholinergic refers to acetylcholine receptors, so *anticholinergic* refers to medications that block acetylcholine). It appears that acetylcholine and dopamine are normally in balance in the part of the brain that controls many involuntary muscle movements. When dopamine is blocked by an antipsychotic medication, this system becomes out of balance and extrapyramidal side effects result. One common way to treat these extrapyramidal side effects is to block acetylcholine, which to some extent restores the dopamine–acetylcholine balance in this part of the brain.

Specifics of Use

Benztropine (Cogentin) is usually prescribed at 1–8 mg/day, often in divided doses. Many people feel that taking the medication once a day is enough, but all antiparkinsonian medications are fairly short-acting, and most people find that they "wear off" if not taken at least twice a day. I usually start with 1 mg once or twice a day, except with elderly people, who need lower doses and with whom much more caution should be taken. On an as-needed basis only, I usually prescribe 2 mg intramuscularly or orally. With severe dystonias or akathisia, the person might be so uncomfortable that intramuscular or intravenous medication is desirable. Other commonly used anticholinergic antiparkinsonian medications include:

- Trihexphenidyl (Artane): usual dose 2–15 mg/day
- Biperiden (Akineton): usual dose 2–8 mg/day

Side Effects

Most antiparkinsonian medications are anticholinergic—that is, they work by blocking the neurotransmitter acetylcholine. As such, they cause the same autonomic side effects as other medications with anticholinergic effects, including clozapine and the older tricyclic antidepressants. These side effects include dry mouth, blurred vision, and constipation. Less frequently, urinary retention, nasal congestion, and muscular weakness become problems. These medications can cause some kinds of glaucoma to worsen or can precipitate glaucoma in people who are already predisposed to develop it.

Finally, all these medications can cause memory and other cognitive impairments, especially in elderly people. These medications can also increase the cognitive problems that are common in many people with schizophrenia. It is important to remember that although these medications make some side effects of the antipsychotic medications better, they make other side effects worse.

These medications are not addictive, but they are sometimes abused. They produce a kind of "altered state" that some people find enjoyable, and as a result they have street value. In higher doses they produce a delirium wherein the person becomes disoriented, loses touch with reality, and sometimes becomes delusional or hallucinates. This delirium can be confused with psychosis. When a person on one of these anticholinergic medications (which include many of the antipsychotics and antidepressants) becomes confused and out of touch with reality, it is important to determine whether he or she is psychotic or delirious.

Diphenhydramine (Benadryl)

Diphenhydramine is a sedating antihistamine that can also be used as a sedative hypnotic (sleeping pill). It also has strong anticholinergic properties that make it useful for treating medication-induced extrapyramidal side effects. Its anticholinergic effects and mild sedation make it particularly useful for treating akathisia in some people. Its effects and side effects are very similar to the other anticholinergic medications.

Amantadine (Symmetrel)

Amantadine has a very different mechanism of action than the other medications used to treat extrapyramidal side effects. The antipsychotic medications all work by blocking the action of dopamine. This dopamine blockade accounts for the beneficial effects of antipsychotics as well as their extrapyramidal side effects. Amantadine works by selectively boosting the action of dopamine, in the part of the brain that is associated with motor side effects. It has minimal effects on dopamine in the part of the brain associated with the therapeutic properties of the antipsychotic medications.

Amantadine has no anticholinergic side effects, and many people tolerate it better than other antiparkinsonian medications. Unfortunately, amantadine is less reliable in the treatment of these motor side effects than are the anticholinergic medications, and it may lose its effectiveness over time in some people.

Occasionally people discontinue amantadine immediately after starting it because they report that it makes them extremely anxious. However, this effect is unusual, and the medication is typically well tolerated. It is now suggested that besides blocking the extrapyramidal side effects of the antipsychotic medications, amantadine may also block other autonomic side effects of the antipsychotics, including weight gain and decreased libido.

Specifics of Use

The usual dose is 100 mg twice/day, which may be increased to 300 mg/day. It takes several days to work.

Beta-Blockers

Beta-blockers are most commonly used to lower high blood pressure, but they also have a large number of other functions. They can decrease the tremors caused by lithium, they can be very is effective in helping a person with performance anxiety, and they may be helpful in other anxiety that has a large somatic component such as sweating and racing pulse. Beta-blockers may also be effective in decreasing rage reactions in some people.

Beta-blockers are exactly what their name says: They block the "beta" epinephrine receptors (epinephrine and adrenaline are different names for the same chemical). Epinephrine is a naturally occurring chemical in the body that is released by nerve cells and the adrenal gland. It stimulates receptor sites on nerve cells, blood vessels, and other parts of the body. Receptors that are stimulated by epinephrine (or its similar first cousin, norepinephrine) are called *adrenergic receptors*. There are two distinct kinds of receptors, alpha-adrenergic and beta-adrenergic receptors. Beta-blockers such as propranolol (Inderal) simply block these beta receptor sites. These occur throughout the body, which partially explains why these medications are used in conditions that seem unrelated. Beta receptors control heart rate, sweating, and other autonomic symptoms. Alpha-adrenergic receptors mediate relaxation of smooth muscle throughout the body, thereby helping to lower blood pressure, decrease urinary retention, and other beneficial effects.

Indications for Use

- *Cardiovascular uses.* Beta-blockers have traditionally been used to help control high blood pressure, treat angina, and control certain kinds of arrhythmias (irregular heartbeats). In addition, beta-blockers are often used to treat migraine headaches, as well as more unusual conditions associated with an outpouring of epinephrine or norepinephrine.
- *Tremors.* Benign tremors respond well to these medications. Beta-blockers in low doses are also very effective in treating a number of different kinds of tremors, including the tremor that is a common side effect of lithium.
- *Performance anxiety.* Beta-blockers are extremely effective in helping people with performance anxiety. The musician or public speaker whose anxiety begins to interfere with his or her performance often has a dramatic response to these medications, used in a very low dose. The anticipatory anxiety before the performance is still there, but the specific performance anxiety can be decreased without any sedation or interference with cognitive or motor abilities. It does not work in the brain but rather decreases the body's response to anxiety—the racing pulse and sweating—which in turn decreases the feedback loop that amplifies the anxiety to levels that interfere with function.
- *Anxiety with marked somatic (physical) symptoms.* Beta-blockers block some of the peripheral symptoms of anxiety. The person may still "think" anxious, but these medications can stop the pounding heart, sweaty palms, tremor, etc., that cause the anxiety to feed upon itself and get out of control. These are most useful as antianxiety agents in people who, in fact, have a lot of somatic manifestations of their anxiety.
- *Akathisia.* Propranolol is also useful as a treatment for akathisia (the motor restlessness caused by antipsychotic medications). Even though akathisia is much less common with the

new atypical antipsychotic medications, it still exists and is still extremely uncomfortable.

- *Violent outbursts.* Some research has suggested that propranolol may be useful in treating certain kinds of violent outbursts, including some of the aggressive behaviors seen in some people with developmental delays. It also may be useful in treating some people with schizophrenia. The dose range is moderate to high—100–2500 mg/day. Using very high doses may be dangerous, although the exact nature of those dangers is somewhat unclear.

- *Prevent the development of PTSD.* The research on this application is still limited, but it does appear that taking a beta-blocker for a few days after a traumatic event may decrease the likelihood that the person will later develop PTSD. The idea is that the beta-blocker interferes with the process that would normally connect the emotional overload to the memory of the event. The actual memory of the event is not impacted, but it may moderate some of the emotional connections. Beta-blockers are not yet recommended for regular use after a traumatic event, but they are safe and well tolerated, and if the research supports early findings, use of this class of medication may become an effective approach to preventing PTSD.

- *Atypical Beta-Blockers.* As was discussed in the beginning of this book, all medications have multiple sites of action. Pindolol (Viskin), an atypical beta-blocker, not only blocks the beta-norepinephrine receptor but also blocks serotonin reuptake (and therefore increases serotonin in the synapse). Whereas most beta-blockers can potentiate depressions, pindolol may increase the effectiveness of SSRIs in treating depression. It might also accelerate the speed of onset of the antidepressants. Unfortunately, the data supporting the use of pindolol in increasing the effectiveness of antidepressants is mixed with some studies supporting its use and a recent study suggesting it does not help. A typical dose is 2.5 mg three times a day. It appears to be less effective with sertraline, probably because of drug–drug interactions.

Specifics of Use

Beta-blockers typically work fairly quickly. Whatever effect a beta-blocker will have will typically manifest within hours of the first dose. This means that these medications can often be taken to control symptoms just when those symptoms are likely to be severe, and may not, in every case, need to be taken every day. Someone taking propranolol or atenolol for performance anxiety can take it a few hours before a speech or performance, and not take it at other times. If the underlying problem is ongoing, such as a lithium tremor, then the treatment may also need to be ongoing. There appears to be little risk or problem with using these medications chronically.

- *Propranolol (Inderal)* is an older beta-blocker and still widely used. It has the most research support for use in anxiety disorders. It is a short-acting medication that sometimes works better if taken twice a day. When used for blood pressure control or for control of irregular heart beats, the dose range is up to 320 mg/day. When used for anxiety or for control of side effects, it is usually started at 10 or 20 mg twice a day, and the total dose is rarely above 80 mg/day. When used for control of aggressive outbursts, higher doses may be required. It also comes in a longer-acting form, Inderal LA.

- *Atenolol (Tenormin)* is a beta-blocker that has a longer period of action than does propranolol. It also has less of a tendency to cross the blood–brain barrier than does propranolol, and may therefore be somewhat less likely to cause psychiatric side effects such as depression. It seems to be as effective as propranolol, but there is less research on its use. It is typically started at 50 mg/day, which can be increased to 100 mg/day if needed.

Side Effects

For the most part, beta-blockers are very safe when used in relatively low doses. They can be dangerous, however, for people with asthma or COPD (chronic obstructive pulmonary disease).

They can also block the clinical recognition of hypoglycemia (low blood sugar). Because people with diabetes may have serious hypoglycemic episodes, the use of beta-blockers with this population can be dangerous.

Beta-blockers can also cause or potentiate depression, especially in the higher doses used to treat high blood pressure and certain cardiac conditions. This effect seems rare even at high doses, however, and very rare in the doses typically used in psychiatric disorders. Beta-blockers can also cause nightmares and a sense of fatigue.

MEDICATIONS FOR PTSD

Trauma of various sorts is very common in our society. There is acute childhood trauma, such as a car accident, or the chronic trauma such as that suffered from ongoing sexual abuse by a trusted adult. There is acute adult trauma such as that after a rape, or the more chronic trauma that comes with prolonged military combat. Although all of these are lumped under the single label of trauma, they are very different from one another in terms of impact and long-term consequences. The data are very imprecise, but the majority of people exposed to severe, life-threatening trauma will experience an acute stress reaction. About 20% of these people will go on to develop more prolonged PTSD. Although it can be permanent, PTSD can also become less intrusive and less bothersome over a period of years. PTSD seems to occur more frequently if the trauma is prolonged, and there is a suggestion that the presence of social support and group cohesion during a trauma may lessen its frequency. Even with prolonged childhood abuse, a particularly type of stressful chronic trauma, usually with no chance for any social support and occurring during the most vulnerable developmental periods, not everyone develops PTSD.

People with PTSD often have flashbacks, during which they can feel that they are back in the midst of the trauma, even years later. Other symptoms, such as nightmares and hypervigilance (a constant sense that the persons needs to be on guard) are also usually present. Situations that can trigger memories or flashbacks, crowds, noisy places, or any environment that has some element that can be connected to the traumatic event, are often avoided. Anger and irritation are common, as is an associated emotional numbness. People with PTSD typically have problems feeling connected to others. These symptoms often cause difficulty in intimate relationships and may cause problems in the workplace. Alcohol or drug abuse is a common complication of living with PTDS.

Psychosocial support seems to be the cornerstone of effective treatment for PTSD. Note that therapies that encourage graphic retelling and reliving of the trauma may actually make PTSD worse, whereas treatments that normalize and support feelings and focus on problem solving and behavior are often useful. A number of medications seem helpful for some of the symptoms of PTSD, although research data are very limited. Many people with PTSD have an associated depression, and SSRI and SNRI antidepressants seem helpful. Other people with PTSD also have symptoms of mood instability, with both "ups" and "downs" cycling very rapidly. A mood stabilizer such as lamotrigine may be useful if the primary symptom is depression. Valproic acid or carbamazepine can also be beneficial in helping to moderate some of the associated mood instability associated with PTSD. Despite the anxiety commonly connected with PTSD, benzodiazepines are not very useful, and dependency and abuse can be a problem.

Medications That Down-Regulate the Adrenergic System

Decreasing activity in the adrenergic system would helps of the symptoms of PTSD, especially the nightmares and hyperarousal. These medications can be a definite help for those people with severe PTSD who respond. Unfortunately, however, less than half of the people with PTSD find medication helpful. If one of these medications is going to be effective, it will usually work within a few days. The medications discussed below all have an FDA indication for the treatment of hypertension.

Alpha-1 Adrenergic Receptor Blockers

Alpha-1 adrenergic receptor blockers block the alpha part of the adrenergic (epinephrine) system. Specifically, they block the alpha-1 receptor, which in turn decreases activity in this system.

Clonidine (Catapres)

Clonidine is normally prescribed for hypertension and benign prostatic hypertrophy (enlarged prostate causing urinary retention). Clonidine was the first medication in this class to demonstrate effectiveness with the nightmares of PTSD. The research on using clonidine in PTSD is still very limited, and although it is used, there is still some controversy about it effectiveness. Clonidine has also been used to help manage the withdrawal symptoms associated with a number of drugs of abuse, from opiates to cocaine.

- *Specifics of use.* Clonidine is usually started at 0.1 mg/day and slowly increased, as needed, up to a maximum of 0.4–0.6 mg/day in divided doses. It is also available as a patch that lasts for 7 days. It generally takes 2–3 days for a person to achieve a full serum level after first applying a patch.
- *Side effects.* The most common side effect is tiredness. Other common side effects include dry mouth, dizziness, constipation, and skin rashes.

Prazosin (Minipress)

Prazosin is normally used for hypertension and benign prostatic hypertrophy (enlarged prostate causing urinary retention). It is now used more frequently than clonidine in PTSD because it is less sedating and causes fewer of the other side effects such as dry mouth.

- *Specifics of use.* It is usually started at 1 mg twice a day, although if sleep disruption is the primary symptom, it can be started 1 or 2 mg all before bed. The dose can be increased up to 6 mg/day.

- *Side effects.* The most common side effects are sedation and blood pressure drops that can cause dizziness or even sudden fainting. Nausea, a sense of general weakness, and headaches are possible but not common. All of these side effects are dose related.

Alpha-Adrenergic Receptor Stimulants (alpha-2 agonist)

Alpha-2 adrenergic receptor agonists stimulate the receptor in adrenergic (epinephrine) system that acts as a brake to "down-regulate" activity.

Guanfacine (Tenex) is commonly used for blood pressure control. It can also be used to decrease some of the discomfort associated with opiate withdrawal, in decreasing some of the intrusive nightmares and flashbacks associated with PTSD—although the research support for this application is limited.

- *Specifics of use.* It is typically started at 1 mg before sleep, and it can be increased up to 3 mg before sleep.
- *Side effects.* Typically sedation, dizziness, dry mouth, and constipation.

MEDICATIONS FOR ATTENTION-DEFICIT/ HYPERACTIVITY DISORDER

ADHD is a disorder of inattention, hyperactivity, and impulsivity. These areas can be broken down further into problems with concentration, sustained attention, regulating alertness, managing frustration, and self-regulation. Sometimes a person can have more of one part of this syndrome and less of another. Although symptoms of ADHD always start in childhood, it is not just a disorder of children, as it often persists into adulthood. The nature of the disorder changes a bit from childhood to adulthood. Adults often have more control over whether they spend long periods of time in a classroom, and they can usually avoid some of the situations that make inattention more difficult. Some symptoms such as hyperactivity tend to decrease over time, whereas the concentration problems often continue. Adult ADHD can cause problems at work and can interfere with family and friends. The concentration problems of ADHD can lead to driving problems and to difficulties in following through with normal day-to-day responsibility.

The problem is that many things can cause concentration difficulties, from depression to anxiety to schizophrenia. Not all concentration problems stem from ADHD. People who are depressed, anxious, or sleepy can all have problems with concentration. It is sometimes very difficult to separate concentration problems related to ADHD from those caused by some other problem. It is the overall pattern of concentration problems that supports the specific diagnosis. ADHD often occurs alongside both substance use and other mental illness, which can make both recognition and treatment more difficult.

A number of assessment scales can be used to make a diagnosis of ADHD, including the Wender Utah Rating Scale (WURS), the Conners Adult Attention/Hyperactivity rating screening scale, and the World Health Organization Adult ADHD self-report scale. Although these rating scales might help, for the most part it is a clinical diagnosis, not one made by numbers on a scale.

A number of medications can be useful in the treatment of ADHD. Stimulants, amphetamines, and methylphenidates increase both norepinephrine and dopamine in the brain, specifically in the frontal area. They are the most effective treatments for ADHD, but they have side effects and are subject to abuse. Atomoxetine (Strattera), a norepinephrine reuptake blocker, and the antidepressant bupropion (Wellbutrin) are both useful, and neither is subject to the abuse of a stimulant, but neither is as effective for as many people as is a stimulant.

Stimulants: Amphetamine and Methylphenidate Preparations

Stimulants—amphetamine (Dexedrine) and methylphenidate (Ritalin)—have had a somewhat checkered career in psychiatry.

There are many situations where stimulants are clearly useful and safe, but they have been so subject to overuse and abuse that many physicians avoid prescribing them. They are under special regulation, and a physician cannot call in a prescription for a stimulant over the phone and cannot mark a prescription to include refills.

In most ways, the various stimulants are more similar than they are different. One may be more effective than another for a specific person or have slightly different side effects. Some have special delivery systems or properties that may make them less subject to abuse.

Indications for Use

ADHD in Children and Adults
The primary indication for the use of stimulants is the treatment of ADHD. These medications can also be useful in the treatment of depression in individuals who have not responded to antidepressants, and in the treatment of narcolepsy. Amphetamines and methylphenidates are most commonly used to treat ADHD in children. Stimulants work paradoxically in children (whether hyperactive or not), helping them calm down and increasing their attention spans. There is no question that amphetamines are helpful in calming hyperactive children; they help these children behave more appropriately at home and in school and enable many of them to stay in normal classes rather than moving to special education. However, there is ongoing debate about whether hyperactivity is overdiagnosed, and whether many of these children would do better with social/psychological, rather than pharmacological, intervention.

In normal adults the effects of these medications are a bit more complicated. If a person is tired and having concentration difficulties because of this fatigue, a stimulant (including caffeine) can increase concentration. If the person is not tired or if too high a dose is taken, concentration will be impaired. The use of stimulants in hyperactive adults is receiving increased attention, although the research is still limited. Adults who have a clear history of childhood hyperactivity (which is often coupled with some history of learning disability or impulsive behavior) and who continue to have very short attention spans may be helped by stimulants.

People with ADHD typically respond rapidly and report a significant improvement in their ability to concentrate and function. This improvement is expressed differently in different people. Some people report that they can concentrate enough to read, whereas before they could not; others report that they can concentrate enough to function better at work or not be so distracted in day-to-day normal activities. In more extreme cases, ADHD can cause significant behavioral disruptions, including fighting and impulsivity, that may decrease with medication. Someone with severe ADHD may take the medication on an ongoing basis, whereas someone with more school- or work-related dysfunction may find that he or she does not need the medication on weekends or on vacation.

Sometimes people respond well to the drug initially but later develop tolerance, so that the medication loses all effect. Within reason, the dose of the medication can be raised or another stimulant can be tried.

Depression
Stimulants also have a role in the treatment of resistant depressions. Most depressed people respond much better to standard antidepressants, but a small number who have not responded to other medications do respond well to small amounts of amphetamine. Use of stimulants is indicated only in unusual situations where there is a clear biological component to the depression, when abuse seems unlikely, and when other somatic treatments have been ineffective. The use of stimulants to treat depression in the elderly has also received renewed attention. Elderly people often have major problems with the side effects of typical antidepressants, and stimulants may be a safe and effec-

tive alternative for some people. Stimulants may also have a special role in treating people who have both depression and serious medical illness, and who have not responded to more traditional approaches.

Narcolepsy

Amphetamines are the treatment of choice with narcolepsy.

Amphetamines

Amphetamines block both the dopamine and norepinephrine reuptake pumps; this blockade keeps more of the neurotransmitters active in the synapse for a longer period than would occur without the medication. Amphetamines also work inside of the neuron to cause the release of extra dopamine into the synapse. This release of dopamine is what makes amphetamines effective in ADHD and depression, and is also what leads to its potential for abuse.

Specifics of Use

There are a number of different amphetamine (and methylphenidate) preparations that vary primarily in their speed of onset and how long they last. There are also some differences in which particular form of amphetamine is used. Shorter-acting medications must be given multiple times a day, whereas longer-acting medications can be given once a day. They are commonly given in the morning or both in the morning and midafternoon, to decrease the problems that they may cause with sleep. There is a very broad dose range of all of these medications, with some people doing very well on a low dose, but other people requiring a much higher dose to achieve a therapeutic effect. For example, the FDA suggests a maximum dose of 60 mg/day for dextroamphetamine, but a higher dose may be required for some people. A need for a higher dose does *not* mean that the medication is being abused.

There are a number of forms of amphetamine products, but the primary compounds include:

- dextroamphetamine (Dexedrine)
- methamphetamine (Desoxyn)
- amphetamine/dextroamphetamine salts (Adderall)

Lisdexamfetamine (Vyvanse) is marketed as a less abusable form of amphetamine. It is a pro-drug that is converted into amphetamine in the body, and it is not effective and does not lead to a "high" if taken intravenously or snorted. It is converted in the GI tract to amphetamine, where it works just as any other amphetamine preparation. It is subject to abuse if taken orally in more than the prescribed dose. It is generally started at 30 mg in the morning and can be increased as necessary.

Side Effects

When taken in very high dose, amphetamines can cause a "high" or rush that some people find extremely pleasurable. Illicit amphetamines are sold as "speed" and "ice," a form of crystalline amphetamine that is extremely pure and very potent. When used in high doses, amphetamines can also cause a paranoid psychosis that can resemble schizophrenia. Even a low dose of amphetamines can cause some individuals to become paranoid. When used in therapeutic doses, amphetamines and other stimulants can cause anxiety, feeling "wired," and agitation. Amphetamines can also cause problems with sleep, loss of appetite, increased blood pressure, and rapid or irregular pulse, and they can worsen tics. There is also concern that the long-term use of stimulants in children may retard normal growth.

Amphetamine-type stimulants have been associated with sudden death in a very small number of both adults and children taking them. Some of these deaths have been associated with people who had preexisting heart problems or who had taken a larger than prescribed dose, but a few of the deaths occurred in people who were taking the medication as directed and who did not have any known heart problems. Table 8.1 lists commonly used amphetamine preparations and their doses and durations.

TABLE 8.1. *Commonly Used Amphetamine Preparations*

	AVERAGE DOSE (MG/DAY)	DURATION (HR.)
Dextroamphetamine (Dexedrine)	10–40	4–9

	AVERAGE DOSE (MG/DAY)	DURATION (HR.)
Dextroamphetamine + amphetamine salts (Adderall)	10–40	5–7
Dextroamphetamine + amphetamine salts, delayed release (Adderall XR)	20–60	10–12
Dextroamphetamine spansules (Dexedrine Spansules)	10–60 mg/day	4–9
Lisdexamfetamine (Vyvanse)		12+

Methylphenidates

Methylphenidates are a stimulant that are very similar to amphetamine, but possibly less addicting and may cause fewer side effects than amphetamine. Like amphetamine, methylphenidate blocks the reuptake of dopamine and norepinephrine back into a nerve cell. Unlike amphetamine, it does not cause the release of dopamine from within the nerve cell.

Methylphenidate is most commonly used to treat attention-deficit disorder (ADD) in both children and adults. The most common side effects are nervousness and insomnia, although nausea, diarrhea, rashes, increased blood pressure, and increased pulse have been reported.

There are a number of different forms of methylphenidate, including slightly different chemical salts, different delivery systems that lead to some that are more long-acting, and even a skin patch.

A typical dose of regular-acting methylphenidate (Ritalin) for adults is 20–40 mg/day, but some people require up to 80 mg/day. It is a short-acting medication and typically must be taken two or three times a day. There is a long-acting form of methylphenidate (Ritalin-SR) that can be given twice a day. The dose of Ritalin-SR is supposed to be the same as regular Ritalin, but anecdotal clinical evidence suggests that a higher dose of the longer-acting preparation may be required to achieve the same effect. The most common forms of methylphenidate include those listed in Table 8.2.

TABLE 8.2. *Commonly Used Methylphenidate Preparations*

	AVERAGE DOSE RANGE (MG)	DURATION OF ACTION (HR.)
Methylphenidate (Ritalin)	10–60	3–5
Methylphenidate extended release (Ritalin LA)	10–60	6–8
Methylphenidate extended release (Ritalin SR)	10–60	4–6
Methylphenidate extended release (Concerta)	10–60	10–12
Methylphenidate extended release (Metadate CD)	10–60	8
Methylphenidate extended release (Metadate ER)	10–60	4–8

Atomoxetine (Strattera)

Atomoxetine is not a stimulant; it is a pure norepinephrine reuptake inhibitor, and it works through a different mechanism than the other medications used for ADHD. Unlike methylphenidate and amphetamine, atomoxetine has no effect on dopamine. This means that atomoxetine does not cause the kind of euphoria that is associated with stimulants. It is a bit less effective, but it has the advantage of having a very low risk of abuse. Atomoextine has a significant advantage if it is prescribed for someone who is at risk for abusing medication, or if there is a significant risk that the medication might be diverted and abused by a family member. It can also be effective in some people with ADHD who have not responded well to the primary stimulants. Despite these advantages in terms of potential for abuse, I generally start with a trial of a primary stimulant over atomoxetine because of the increased efficacy of the older medications, except when abuse is a significant concern.

Atomoxetine has been considered for use as an antidepressant, but it did not seem effective in trials. However, it has been used to augment the effectiveness of SSRI antidepressants. Theoretically the combination of atomoxetine plus an SSRI should work, but the available data have not indicated any significant advantage for the combination or an SSRI alone.

Specifics of Use
Atomoxetine is usually started in adults at 40 mg in the morning, increasing after a few days to 80 mg if needed. Maximum dose is usually 100 mg/day.

Side Effects
Common side effects of atomoxetine include dry mouth, heartburn, nausea, and sleep problems. It has also been associated with decreased appetite, constipation, urinary retention, tiredness, increased sweating, and sexual problems. More serious problems include angio-edema (rapid swelling of skin and mucosal membranes, which can cause breathing difficulty), increased psychotic symptoms, and increased pulse and blood pressure. There is a black box warning from the FDA that it can cause an increase in suicidal behavior.

Modafanil (Provigil)
Modafanil is a stimulant that works through a very different mechanism of action than the other stimulants. It is a histamine agonist; that is, it stimulates histamine receptors. Antihistamines, typically used for treatment of allergies or colds, are generally sedating. Histamine is an activating system, and things that block it are sedating. Medications that increase histamine activity are activating. Because it does not directly stimulate dopamine, modafanil is much less subject to abuse than other stimulants and is less likely to cause psychotic symptoms.

Indications for Use
Modafanil is FDA approved for the sleepiness connected with narcolepsy, sleep apnea, and shift work. It is useful for ADHD but concerns over the risk of Stevens–Johnson syndrome kept the FDA from approving it for this use. It can also be useful

in decreasing the sedative side effects of clozapine and similar medications. It may be helpful to augment the effectiveness of antidepressants in some people who have not responded to other medication combinations.

Specifics of Use
Modafinil is available in 100 and 200 mg tablets. Some people respond well to 50 mg, so I start with ½ a tablet, then increase the dose every few days as needed. Most people respond by 200 mg/day, but the dose can be raised to 400 mg/day if needed. It is long-acting and can be given once a day in the morning.

Side Effects
The biggest concern is the very rare risk of Stevens–Johnson syndrome. This often, but not always, begins with a simple rash and then proceeds to a very serious rash that can be very dangerous. Rashes are more likely to be dangerous if they involve larger areas of the chest or face, or if they involve the surface of the hands or feet. Any fever with swelling of lymph glands should be taken seriously, and if the rash is accompanied by a fever and swollen lymph glands, it should be taken very seriously. Other side effects of modafinil include increased or engendered psychotic symptoms, headache, nausea, runny nose, anxiety, and dry mouth.

MEDICATIONS TO TREAT ALZHEIMER'S DISEASE

There are now two different classes of medications that are useful in the treatment of Alzheimer's disease. *Anticholinesterase* inhibitors increase the amount of acetylcholine in the brain. *NMDA antagonists* block the effect of the activating neurotransmitter glutamate. Both can improve some of the cognitive symptoms of Alzheimer's disease, but the effects are modest and it does not appear that either class of medication affects the ongoing course of the illness. It is likely that in the near future medications will be available that will actually change the course of the disease, but at this time such medications are not available.

Anticholinesterase Inhibitors

Although Alzheimer's disease affects many different neurotransmitter systems in the brain, acetylcholine seems to be particularly impacted. It has been found that medications that decrease or block acetylcholine tend to impair memory. All of the anticholinergic medications used to treat Parkinson's disease or parkinsonian antipsychotic side effects cause some degree of memory impairment. This impairment is worse in older people or people who already have some degree of deficit, but it is measurable even in younger people. All medications that increase acetylcholine activity in the brain tend to improve memory, at least in people with Alzheimer's disease and perhaps in other people as well. Until recently there was no way of easily and safely increasing acetylcholine in the brain. As a group, the medications that do have this ability work by blocking acetylcholinesterase, the main enzyme that breaks apart and deactivates acetylcholine.

Although these medications seem to improve current function, they will not prevent or reverse the eventual deterioration seen in Alzheimer's disease. It seems that they can delay cognitive loss and help to maintain function. They are most effective in people with mild to moderate dementia, although recent data suggest that they can be helpful in people with more severe illness as well. In the United States it is generally recommended that people start on an anticholinesterase inhibitor as soon as a diagnosis of Alzheimer's disease is made. It appears that people started on these medications earlier in their illness experience better functioning than people started later on the same medications. The research is complicated; it should be noted that in England these medications are not recommended for routine use.

Some people respond very well to these medications, which very significantly slow the course of their illness and, to some extent even reverse some of the already existing cognitive deficits. Other people have a more modest response. Whereas a higher does of an anticholinesterase inhibitor can lead to more side effects, primarily nausea, a higher dose is also more likely to lead to a better response over time. If the person can tolerate the side effects, he or she is more likely to have a better response if taking the medication at the upper end of the dose range. Three anticholinesteras inhibitors are available:

1. Donepezil (Aricept) is the oldest of these medications. Starting at a lower dose and increasing the dose slowly leads to fewer GI side effects. It is typically started at 5 mg/day and increased over several weeks to 10 mg/day.
2. Rivastigmine (Exelon) is shorter-acting, so it should be taken twice a day. It is started at 1.5 mg twice a day and increased to 3–6 mg twice a day. It is generally better tolerated if taken with food. It is also available as a daily patch for people who find swallowing a pill difficult.
3. Galantamine (Razadyne, previously called Reminyl) has been found to both decrease the rate of decline of memory and other cognitive functions, and may improve memory in mild dementia. It is usually started at 4 mg twice a day with food, and slowly increased to 12 mg twice a day.

Side Effects

All of the newer cognitive enhancers have very similar side effects, based on their mechanism of action of increasing acetylcholine. About half of the people taking these medications experience nausea, and nausea is the most common reason that people discontinue the medication. Taking the medication with food can help to limit the GI side effects. Other side effects are less common and include vomiting, diarrhea, dizziness, headache, and fatigue. These side effects can be decreased by starting the medication at a lower dose and building up the dose more slowly.

NMDA Antagonist

NMDA receptors are among the major receptors that are stimulated by glutamate, the primary activating neurotransmitter in the brain. Glutamate is present in large amounts throughout the brain, and it probably impacts many other psychiatric disorders, including depression and schizophrenia. Precise regulation is important, since too much glutamate activity can overstimulate nerve cells and lead to nerve cell death.

Memantine (Namenda) is currently the only NMDA receptor antagonist available. It seems to work by decreasing some of the cell death that is associated with Alzheimer's disease. It does not appear to work on the primary cause of the illness, but it does help to decrease some of the secondary damage. It can be used in combination with any of the anticholinesterase medications.

- Specifics of use: Memantine is usually started at 5 mg/day and increased by 5 mg per week up to 10 mg twice a day.
- Side effects: Memantine is generally well tolerated, although it can cause some dizziness, headache, confusion, or constipation. In rare cases it can cause tiredness, hallucinations, GI problems, or shortness of breath.

MEDICATIONS TO TREAT ALCOHOL DEPENDENCE AND SUBSTANCE ABUSE

The most effective approach to the treatment of substance abuse is integrated drug–alcohol treatment that includes education and group and individual therapy. Key ideas are those from motivational interviewing, which stages treatment to start with where the client is "at" and then encourages a commitment to change. Elements of effective treatment usually include education about substance use, relapse prevention strategies, changing environments to support sobriety, and skill training to better cope with situations that traditionally led to substance use. Groups, either professionally led or 12-step types, are often an important part of an effective treatment package. Attention to trauma and loss are typically important. The active treatment of other comorbid mental health problems, weather depression, bipolar disorder, panic disorder, or schizophrenia, can also help a person reassert control over his or her substance use. In addition, there are an increasing array of medications that can help as part of integrated treatment. Medication can be an important part of treatment for some people, but it should never be the primary focus of substance use treatment.

Medications for Alcohol Abuse

There are now four pharmacological approaches to helping people decrease problem drinking; (1) disulfiram (Antabuse), (2) naltrexone (ReVia), (3) acamprosate (Campral), and (4) topiramate (Topamax).

Disulfiram (Antabuse)

Disulfiram makes it impossible for people to drink because they get very sick if they ingest alcohol within a few days of taking the medication. This means that a person who decides to drink while taking disulfiram must wait up to a week or more before actually taking the first drink. For some people, this period of enforced reflection is extremely useful. Disulfiram can be extremely useful for patients who want to stop drinking but feel that they cannot control their impulsive use of alcohol.

Disulfiram has significant limitations, however. Many patients refuse to take it or go off it to resume drinking. Some patients can drink even while taking disulfiram, either because they become less ill or because they can get drunk enough to not feel the discomfort caused by the medication. A full disulfiram–alcohol reaction can be dangerous, especially in someone with other serious medical problems, particularly heart disease. Many patients can get a disulfiram–alcohol reaction from cough medicine or even mouthwash containing alcohol. In addition, disulfiram has other significant drug–drug interactions; for example, it can increase the serum level of commonly used medications, such as phenytoin (Dilantin). Disulfiram's side effects include liver disease, rashes, tiredness, headaches, and, at times, psychosis. These side effects are dose related and are less frequent if the dose is kept at 250 mg/day.

Naltrexone (ReVia)

Naltrexone blocks natural opiate receptors in the brain. It has been used for many years to block the euphoric effects of drugs such as heroin. It is now clear that it can also decrease alcohol craving and significantly increase abstinence when it is used as part of a comprehensive alcohol treatment program. The initial research on naltrexone extended for 3–6 months, and initially it was suggested that the medication should be discontinued after 6 months. Although there is concern about increasing risk of liver damage with long-term use, some people are much more likely to maintain their sobriety if they continue to use naltrexone for a longer period of time.

Naltrexone will both decrease craving and decrease the sense of pleasure that comes with alcohol use. As a result, even if a person does relapse, he or she will be much more likely to have a drink or two and then stop instead of proceeding to a much more destructive out-of-control binge.

It has been suggested that naltrexone may decrease self-injurious behavior and other kinds of compulsive-type behavior. There are scattered reports of using naltrexone to ameliorate the self-abuse in which some people with developmental delays engage. There is also a report of using it in pathological gambling.

Naltrexone precipitates sudden, very uncomfortable withdrawal in anyone who has recently used any opiate such as heroin or morphine. Before starting the medication, patients should be asked about opiate use, and the risk of withdrawal should be explained. There is also some risk of liver damage, especially at larger doses and perhaps when used over a longer period of time. Naltrexone is usually well tolerated, but it can cause insomnia, anxiety, abdominal pain, nausea, and decreased energy in some patients.

A typical dose is 50 mg/day. There is concern about liver problems if the dose it increased beyond this level. Naltrexone is now available as a monthly injection called Vivitrol. This is an effective strategy for some people who find naltrexone useful but are not consistent about taking the pill.

Acamprosate (Campral)

Acamprosate decreases the withdrawal effects of alcohol. It turns out that there are withdrawal "twinges," often triggered by events or places, which can increase the risk of relapse.

Blocking these withdrawal effects seems to help prevent such a relapse. It used to be thought that a person was fully withdrawn from alcohol after a few days or at most weeks of abstinence. It now appears that getting the brain back in balance takes much longer, months at least, and that there are elements of withdrawal that can trigger relapse during this time. Acamprosate may decrease some of this discomfort and decrease the likelihood that a trigger will lead to relapse. Acamprosate probably works by restoring balance between GABA, the major inhibitory system in the brain, and glutamate, the major excitatory system in the brain.

Acamprosate seems most effective when started after a person has achieved at least a few days of sobriety. The data suggest that acamprosate has a modest rather than an overwhelming effect—and it requires that the person swallow a lot of pills: An effective dose is two pills three times a day. It is generally well tolerated, although headache, flatulence, diarrhea, and nausea have been reported.

Topiramate (Topamax)

Topiramate is an anticonvulsant that causes weight loss. It was investigated as a potential mood stabilizer, but several well-done trials did not find it to be effective for this purpose (see also Chapter 6). Some studies have suggested that topiramate may be useful in helping to decrease both days drinking and heavy drinking days in men with alcohol dependence, and that it may be helpful in cocaine dependence, although this cocaine-related research is still very preliminary. So far there are no studies looking at the effect of topiramate on women with alcohol dependence. There are also some data that topiramate may decrease self-injurious behavior in people diagnosed with borderline personality disorder.

Topiramate can have significant cognitive side effects, the most common of which is a problem with word finding (coming up with a specific name or word). It can also cause problems with concentration, confusion, dizziness, and tiredness. These side effects can be minimized by starting topiramate at a low dose, 25 mg/day, and increasing the dose every few days. Topiramate can also cause metabolic acidosis, a rare but serious side effect. Symptoms include hyperventilation, significant fatigue, and nausea.

Medications for Opiate Dependence

Methadone

Methadone is a long-acting opiate that is used both for control of severe pain and for treatment of heroin and other opiate addiction. Since it is a long-acting medication, it causes less of the highs and lows than does heroin, and since it can be given legally in certified methadone clinics, it allows a person to stabilize his or her life even while staying dependent on an opiate. A sufficient dose of methadone blocks many of the opiate receptors, and someone taking methadone will find heroin less reinforcing than without methadone. Unfortunately methadone itself is subject to abuse. It is available only for treatment of addiction within very tightly regulated, specially certified clinics. It initially requires that a person come to the clinic daily to take that day's dose of methadone, and even after significant stability the number of doses that can be dispensed at a time is very tightly controlled.

Buphrenorphine/Naloxone (Suboxone)

Buphrenorphine is a significant breakthrough in the treatment of people with opiate addiction. As a partial opiate agonist, buphrenorphine This means that it both blocks opiate receptors in the brain and also weakly stimulates those same receptors. In the process, it blocks the effect of heroin and other opiates, and is considerably less subject to abuse than a pure opiate agonist such as methadone. A person taking buphrenorphine will not feel any high or other effect if he or she takes a dose of heroin or some other opiate. Without the reinforcing effect, the opiate use pattern is much easier to control. Combining buphrenorphine in a preparation with naloxone, which is a potent opiate blocker, means that if a person tries to inject the medication instead of taking it orally, it will block, rather than stimulate, opiate receptors, further decreasing the risk of abuse. Because the abuse potential is fairly low, it can be given in a clinic with much less regulation than methadone, and it can be dispensed for a longer period of time so a person is not tied to coming into the clinic for a daily dose of medication. It seems effective and well tolerated. It can only be prescribed by physicians who have gone through a special training program.

Medications for Smoking Cessation

Two medications have now been shown to help people quit smoking when used in conjunction with a behavioral program focused on quitting. These can both be used in conjunction with nicotine replacement (gum, patch, or inhaler) and can used together as well.

Bupropion (Wellbutrin, Zyban)

Bupropion, which is primarily used as an antidepressant, can provide some additional help to people who are trying to stop smoking and are engaged in a stop smoking program. It seems to work even for people who are not depressed. Among the antidepressants, this ability to help a person stop smoking is limited to bupropion: Other antidepressants are not effective for this use. Zyban and Wellbutrin are different names for bupropion, which is also available as a generic product.

Varenicline (Chantix)

Varenicline blocks nicotine receptors in the brain, which in turn blocks some of the reinforcing effects of cigarettes, making quitting easier. It is most effective when used along with a stop smoking program, and it can be used in addition to bupropion. It is probably more effective than bupropion, but even so, less than half the people in studies were able to quit smoking even with the varenicline. Support for not smoking is critical. It is also important to keep trying. Often people are not able to stop smoking the first or second time they try, but eventually they achieve it.

The most common side effects of varenicline are problems with sleep, constipation, nausea, or gas. There have also been reports of an increase in depression and even suicidal thoughts while taking this medication. It can be used in people with a history of depression or other mental illness, but the person and his or her support system should be alert for any changes in mood.

9

Medication for People with Borderline Personality Disorder

As discussed at the beginning of this book, medications are tools that people can use to overcome the symptoms and disabilities caused by their mental illness. The relationship between the person taking the medication and the person prescribing the medication is critically important. This relationship greatly affects whether the assessment will be accurate, whether the medication will be taken, and whether the medication is seen as a tool or just one more way that the person labeled "client" or "patient" has lost control over his or her life. The prescriber must be technically knowledgeable about the medication, but must also be skilled and interested in establishing a healing and trusting relationship. This principle holds true throughout psychiatry and medicine, but it is particularly true when working with people who have difficulty in establishing and maintaining stable relationships.

Many books have been written about people diagnosed with borderline personality disorder, and more will come in the future. There are disagreements about the nature of the disorder, the cause, and certainly the treatment. One area where there is widespread agreement is that this diagnosis is applied to people who have unstable relationships. This relational instability is, in fact, the core problem that leads to the diagnosis. Medications can be very effective tools for people with this diagnosis, but only if the relationship issues are attended to first. There is nothing in this section that would not apply to anyone taking medication; it is just that issues in the relationship are most likely to interfere with the effective use of medication in this population.

I have spoken with many people who have a borderline diagnosis who tell me that medications do not work for them. They have been on fluoxetine (Prozac) for a week, Zoloft for 2 days, risperidone for 3 days, and divalproex (Depakote) for 2 weeks, and none of them worked. They often feel frustrated by their attempts to work with a prescriber and desperate for something that will help them deal with their pain and chaos, hoping that medication might be an answer. At the same time, they are often noncompliant, using medications in ways that allows little chance of success.

A "personality disorder" is not a symptom as much as a way of living in the world. It is a pervasive, persistent, maladaptive behavior pattern that affects many areas of the person's life. We all have different ways of protecting ourselves from stress and from perceived threats. We all have bits and pieces of effective as well as maladaptive behavior. People with a personality disorder protect themselves in ways that cause overwhelming and recurrent problems for themselves and for those around them.

OVERVIEW OF BORDERLINE PERSONALITY DISORDER

Any label gives very incomplete information. A particular diagnosis, including that of borderline personality disorder, does not tell us anything about whether or not a person is smart, creative, generous, artistic, or all of the other attributes and strengths that are important to who we are. Diagnosis is shorthand; it describes a small number of attributes that seem to fall into a pattern. Some of the criteria that go into having a diagnosis of borderline personality disorder include the following from the fourth edition, recised, of the *Diagnostic Manual of Mental Disorders* (DSM-IV-TR; American Psychiatric Association, 2000):
• Avoidance of abandonment
• Unstable, intense interpersonal relationships
• Identity disturbance, unstable self-image/sense of self

- Potentially self-damaging impulsiveness
- Recurrent suicidal or self-mutilating behavior
- Affective instability
- Chronic feelings of emptiness or boredom
- Inappropriate anger
- Transient paranoid ideation or severe dissociative symptoms

Not everyone with this diagnosis has all of these symptoms, but the overall sense is of someone who lives a life of chronic crisis and interpersonal instability. At the same time, people with a borderline diagnosis may have many skills and areas of competence. They may be extremely bright and creative, and may excel in work. Overall, however, their life is far from what they would like it to be.

Core Deficits

I find it useful to think about the underlying problems experienced by people with borderline personality disorder. There are many different lists of "core deficits," but I think of them as the following:

- *Affective instability.* The person switches from being depressed to being happy to being suicidal, often rapidly and without clear reason. For many people with this diagnosis, this volatility has been part of their experience since early childhood. The disorder probably has a large biological component that leads to a sense of not being able to trust one's own feelings, since they change unpredictably.
- *Sense of self as being damaged/defective/not good.* The majority of people with borderline personality disorder have had a history of recurrent, often prolonged, sexual abuse. Others have had other kinds of invalidating experiences. Not all people with this diagnosis have had these kinds of horrific childhood experiences, and many people with sexual abuse or other invalidating experiences do not develop a borderline disorder. Whatever the nature of the experience, most people with borderline personality disorder grow up feeling that there is something wrong with them, that they do not fit

in anywhere, and that they are damaged or defective in some fundamental way.

- *Difficulty maintaining their own sense of identity.* This difficulty follows from the first two problems. If you have a constantly changing mood, you learn that you cannot trust your own feelings. If you also experience recurrent abuse from someone who is supposed to protect you, you learn that you cannot trust the outside world either. It is easy to imagine how without either internal or external anchors, one can feel defective, confused, and lost, with no sense of self.

- *Impulsiveness and low frustration tolerance.* Impulsiveness and problems dealing with frustration seem to follow automatically for many people with the other core deficits. Our sense of self, our feeling of competency, our belief that we can stay in control, all aid us as we cope with day-to-day frustrations. These beliefs in one's own ability are often lacking in people with a borderline diagnosis. There is also a significant genetic/biological component to impulsivity, which means that some people are more biologically prone to impulsive beahvior, and will have more difficulty learning to overcome their biological predisposition.

Medication will not correct all of the issues that people with this disorder face, but it can provide help with specific symptoms. For example, medication can help with affective lability as well as some of the anxiety, depression, and impulsiveness that are all common problems faced by people with this disorder. The problem is that at best, medications can only help parts of the problem, and they must be used consistently to have any positive effect.

Effective help for someone with borderline personality disorder requires a nonblaming approach that starts from the premise that the person's problems are caused by a lack of necessary skills, and that these skills can be learned. The issue is not one of a "bad" or unmotivated person, but of someone who is unable—because of skill deficits, biological issues, or personal trauma—to control his or her behavior. This brief chapter does not attempt to provide a comprehensive overview on the treatment of people with borderline personality disorder, but some ideas about treatment are necessary to set a context in which medication can be useful. It is difficult to prescribe for a person who is impulsive, angry, and tends to have major issues with control. Medication only has a chance of actually being taken and being effective if used within a stable and caring clinical relationship.

Therapeutic Assumptions

Behaviorally oriented psychotherapy is the foundation of effective treatment for people with borderline personality disorder. The best-researched and best-known treatment approach is that associated with Marsha Linehan. Medications can assist psychotherapy in some cases, but it is the therapy that is the core of treatment. Dialectical behavior therapy, as described by Linehan, outlines a set of assumptions and approaches that seem as useful in structuring a medication trial as they are in structuring psychotherapy (closely adapted from Linehan):

1. *People with BPD (borderline personality disorder) are doing the best they can.*
   - People with BPD want to improve.
   - People with BPD need to do better, try harder, and be more motivated to change.
   - People with BPD may not have caused all of their own problems, but they have to solve them anyway.
   - The lives of suicidal, borderline individuals are unbearable as they are currently being lived.
   - People with BPD must learn new behaviors in all relevant contexts.
   - People with BPD cannot fail in therapy.
2. *Therapists treating people with BPD need support.*
   - The goal is to stay in a long term, stable relationship.
   - Know the limits of your responsibility.
   - Be aware of your own feelings.
   - Monitor and regulate interpersonal distance.

- Be aware of "splitting"—being "right" may be less important than being a team.
- Be clear about the therapy contract.

Before Starting a Medication Trial

Before starting a medication trial with a person who has a borderline personality disorder diagnosis, some basic information needs to be collected. Medication is a tool that is more likely to be useful if both the person taking the medication and the person prescribing the medication are clear about what they want it to accomplish.

A.   What does the person prescribed the medication want?
- What are the person's treatment goals?
- What would "doing better" or "doing worse" look like? Be concrete and specific.
- What commitment is the person willing and able to make?

B.   What do you want as the prescriber?
- What are you able to deliver? Do not promise more than you can provide.
- What can you not tolerate? Do not agree to something that you cannot continue to support (e.g., receiving emergency phone calls at home, or not sharing critical information with other members of the treatment team).
- What behaviors would make it difficult for you to continue the relationship?
- How much risk can you tolerate? How far are you able to go in supporting the person?

C.   Obtain a careful history.
1. Assess the person's strengths.
   - How has the person managed to survive in his or her chaotic world?
   - In what areas has the person developed resiliency?
   - Where does the person get support?
   - When has the person done well?: What have been the

person's stablest relationship, best job, and best period of function?

2. Consider that the person's problematic behaviors are exacerbated by:
   • Treatable medical illness
   • Coexisting mental illness
   • Sequela of trauma
   • Substance abuse
3. Review pharmacological treatment carefully and in detail.
   • What medications have been tried?
   • How much for how long?
   • What has worked, even a little?
   • What has not worked?
   • What has been tried but discontinued quickly? What side effects were particularly bothersome?

ELEMENTS OF A MEDICATION TRIAL

• *Develop a collaborative relationship with shared treatment goals BEFORE starting any medication.* If this basic step cannot be accomplished, it is highly unlikely that medication will be used or useful. Spend as much time as necessary, over multiple sessions or even multiple months, developing a collaborative relationship. A corollary of this principle is that the prescriber should never want a person with a borderline diagnosis to take medication more than the person him- or herself wants the medication. Trying too hard to "sell" or coerce medication is highly likely to lead to control fights rather than effective treatment.

• *Identify specific target symptoms.* For example, a person who is now suicidal much of the time may have a goal of feeling less suicidal. The important next step is to be concrete about what this "less" would look like. If the person currently feels suicidal several times a day, feeling suicidal only once a day would be an improvement.

• *Discontinue medication if target symptoms do not improve.*

The hardest part of prescribing is not starting a new medication; it is stopping an old one even if it was not effective. An individual taking a medication often feels that it is doing "something," and is reluctant to stop. Similarly, staff may be concerned that the person will be even worse without it. As a result it is easy for people with a diagnosis of borderline personality disorder to end up on a list of multiple medications, none of which is working very well but all of which are potentially causing side effects.

- *Medication decisions are never an emergency.* People with a diagnosis of borderline personality disorder often lead chaotic lives of chronic crisis. They may call feeling desperate that something must be done NOW, that the medication decision cannot wait for reflection, education, and joint planning. Medications all take some time to work. If it really is a crisis, the medication will not work fast enough to help anyway. The role of medication is to help the person stabilize his or her life, but medication is highly unlikely to be an effective response to crisis unless it is part of an agreed-upon and carefully considered plan.

- *Patient education is critical.* The entire approach to people with a borderline diagnosis is to help them develop new skills, new coping capacities, and new ways of dealing with the world. Having as much information as possible about medication or any other tools being employed will help the person use those tools more effectively.

- *Get clear agreement on what medication, for how long.* I often see people who have had multiple ineffective medication trials, often accompanied by significant side effects and significant difficulty tolerating those side effects long enough to see if the medication will do any good. I try very hard to help the person make a plan for coping with the time it will take to see if the medication will really work, and I seek to elicit a commitment that the person will try and stay on the medication for that entire period of time. If the person is unable to give such a commitment, I wait to start the medication trial until we have enough trust with each other that a commitment can be made.

MEDICATIONS IN BORDERLINE PERSONALITY DISORDER

There is very little controlled research to provide a guide about how medications should be used in people with borderline disorder, and none of the medications discussed below have an FDA indication for their use in this population. Even more than in the other sections of this book, the information on using medication who have people with a diagnosis of borderline personality disorder is based on my own experience, with relatively little guidance from the research literature. The biological understanding of the disorder is still very limited. There are no medications for "borderline," per se, but there are medications that are useful for the symptoms of the disorder. As a result, I focus medication on specific symptoms without worrying too much about theory or cause. The same medications used in other areas of psychiatry are used with people who have borderline disorder. If someone is depressed, I consider an antidepressant. If someone becomes disorganized under stress, I consider an antipsychotic. There are, however, some guidelines about how these medications should be used in people with borderline disorder.

Mood Stabilizers

Since mood instability is part of the core problem of borderline personality disorder, mood stabilizers would seem to be the cornerstone of treatment for many people with this disorder. Even people who complain of severe and even suicidal depressions often have a cyclical course to their mood, with periods of relatively better feeling interspersed with periods of feeling worse. If the depression is treated directly with an antidepressant, there is a risk of increasing the intensity and frequency of these mood swings. My clinical experience suggests that mood stabilizers can be very useful, but the controlled research is extremely limited and results have not been consistently positive. The three medications I have used for this disorder are:

- Divalproex sodium (Depakote)
- Carbamazepine (Tegretol)
- Oxcarbazepine (Trileptal)

The best research support is for divalproex sodium, which decreases anger and interpersonal sensitivity but not depression. Weight gain can be a side effect of divalproex sodium, and it can become large enough to be a significant problem for some people taking it. My experience suggests that lithium is probably less useful in this population, and I will typically start with a trial of divalproex (Depakote). All three of these medications can also help to decrease impulsiveness, and increase "reflective delay." Although clinically I find it useful, the research support for the effectiveness of carbamazepine (Tegretol) is mixed. It does not cause the weight gain associated with divalproex, but its other side effects are often more difficult to live with, and it has a bit more risk in its use. Oxcarbazepine is a metabolite (breakdown product) of carbamazepine that is safer and has fewer side effects than does the parent medication, but it is unclear if it is as effective. One study suggested it was effective in the dose range of 1200–1500 mg/day, but it is always hard to interpret the significance of findings from a single study.

The dose range of all of these medications is much broader in people with a borderline diagnosis than when the same medications are used in people with a bipolar disorder. Some people with a borderline disorder do very well with doses of medication that would be thought to be too low to be effective. On the other hand, other people need a full dose. "Starting low and going slow" is the normal procedure. By starting at a very low dose and increasing it much more slowly than normal, it is possible to see results at lower dose levels, if they are going to occur, and side effects are decreased by the slower increase.

The goal is to "even out" some of the mood instability without causing too many side effects or too much emotional blunting or flattening. Careful attention to dose can help this process.

Lamotrigine (Lamictal)

The other available mood stabilizers are more effective on the "up" side of the mood instability. Lamotrigine is the first mood stabilizer that has shown efficacy in the "down" or depressed side of the instability continuum. It must be started at a low dose and increased very slowly because of the risk of rash. As a result, it takes months to get up to an effective dose. Although lamotrigine is not immediately useful, it is well worth trying in someone with mood instability for whom the depression is a major problem. It also seems useful in helping some people with borderline disorder control their reactive anger.

Topiramate (Topamax)

There are now two well-done studies suggesting that topiramate can help people with borderline disorder decrease chronic self-destructive behavior such as cutting. Topiramate is attractive because it causes weight loss rather than weight gain, and obesity is often a frequent concern. It is not effective as a mood stabilizer and has a number of significant side effects, such as word-finding difficulties. Specifically, topiramate can make it more difficult to rapidly think up a specific word or name. Some people seem to do well on topiramate with few side effects, whereas others find it difficult to tolerate.

Gabapentin (Neurontin)

The available research data on gabapentin suggest that it is not generally useful for people with bipolar disorder. On the other hand, there is anecdotal experience that it can be useful for some people with rapid mood cycles or mood instability. As a result it is commonly tried in people with borderline disorder. As with other medications, it is not always helpful, but some individuals do respond remarkably well to this medication. It is generally well tolerated with relatively few side effects for most people, although can cause sedation and weight gain, especially when used at a higher dose. It is useful in the pain associated with fibromyalgia and the pain associated with diabetes and other illnesses that damage nerves.

Pregabalin (Lyrica)

Pregabalin is a newer (and more expensive) medication that seems similar to gabapentin in both action and effectiveness. It may cause less sedation and less weight gain than gabapentin. There are very few data on the use of pregabalin in any psychiatric condition.

(See Chapter 6 for more information about mood stabilizers.)

Antidepressants

Traditionally, antidepressants are the medications first prescribed for people with borderline personality disorder, and virtually all of the patients whom I see with this diagnosis have already had at least one trial of an SSRI or other antidepressant. Clinically the SSRI/SNRIs seem useful for some people, perhaps be somewhat more so for impulsive aggression. The modest findings of improvement in the few controlled research studies that are available suggest that the results are likely to be modest for many people. There is even less research on the use of bupropion or mirtazapine, both of which seem useful in some people, based on my experience and anecdotal reports. In particular, bupropion tends to increase energy without significant weight gain or sexual side effects, whereas mirtazapine is very sedating, helps regularize sleep, and seems useful for its anti-anxiety/anti-panic properties as well as for its antidepressant effects. All of these newer medications have the advantage of being much safer than the older medications that they replaced. Although any overdose can be dangerous, an overdose is much less likely to be lethal with one of the newer antidepressants.

With development of many newer, safer, and better-tolerated antidepressants, MAOIs are now rarely prescribed, although they can still be an important part of treatment for people who have not responded to other antidepressants. There are better data for the effectiveness of MAOIs than any other class of antidepressant, but these drugs are difficult to prescribe, have many side effects and dietary restrictions involving many common foods. Furthermore, MAOIs are dangerous in overdose and have a significant number of serious drug–drug interactions. Having said all of this about their danger and inconvenience, at times they can be very effective. MAOIs can be used only with someone who has been very well educated on both the risks and benefits of the medication, and who can follow all of the required restrictions. Emsam (selegiline transdermal) is an MAOI that comes in a skin patch instead of a pill. It bypasses the gut and therefore does not require food restrictions, although the drug–drug interactions continue to be a concern.

People with borderline personality often seem much more sensitive to side effects. There is also concern that antidepressant increase the emotional instability of someone who may already have problematic ups and downs in his or her mood. For all of these reasons, I would again suggest starting these medications at somewhat less than normal doses and increasing a bit more slowly than one would with someone who has a more straightforward depression.

It is very important to reinforce the value of developing a very clear patient–clinician collaboration about the use of the medication before starting it. The target symptoms should be clearly laid out, and the likely time that it will take the person to know whether or not the medication is going to work. Attempts should be made to avoid starting a medication that is likely to be stopped in a few days or when the person taking the medication is unlikely to agree to increase to an effective dose.

Very often, the first and the second medication do not work, but then the third medication tried turns out to be very useful. People often respond to one of the antidepressants but not another. There is no way to predict this response, which means that a trial-and-error process is sometimes required. (See Chapter 5 for more information about antidepressants.)

Antipsychotics

An antipsychotic medication, typically in a very low dose, is often very useful in helping people with a borderline diagnosis organize their thoughts. The second-generation antipsychotic medications are better tolerated and may be more effective than the older medications. They are less likely than the first-generation antipsychotic medications to cause extrapyramidal side effects, and are much less likely to cause tardive dyskinesia. Finally, they appear to work better as mood stabilizers than the older antipsychotic medications. On the other hand, some of the second-generation antipsychotic medications may cause significant weight gain.

As with any medication trials, it is critical to have specific target symptoms identified for each person before starting a medication. Antipsychotic medications can be used to target anxiety, mood instability, brief psychotic episodes, thought disorganization, and hyperactivity.

Many people with borderline disorder go through periods of severe anxiety. Often they can become disorganized during these periods, with trouble concentrating and focusing. This anxiety often has a different feel from normal anxiety, and is often accompanied by significant distress. At times, people with borderline personality disorder develop mini-psychotic episodes, with some short-lived psychotic symptoms.

Antipsychotic medications can reduce this anxiety and help people organize their thinking and feel less scattered. Although there are some risks and side effects associated with the second-generation antipsychotic medications, they are not addictive and not generally abused. They are also relatively safe if they are taken in an overdose.

Specifics of Use

Almost always, very low doses of antipsychotic medication are both effective and well tolerated. Doses that would be ineffective in people with schizophrenia are often very useful in people with borderline disorder. Often, higher, more "normal," doses of these medications are less useful and produce more side effects. In particular, people with borderline disorder often feel "blunted" if the dose of the medication is raised too much.

People with borderline disorder often find that their antipsychotic medication can be taken only when needed, rather than in the same dose every day. Again, this is very different from the way in which these same medications are used by people with schizophrenia. For some people, antipsychotic medications can be a tool that help them cope with stress without feeling so overwhelmed. Again, they do not work for everyone with a borderline disorder, but they may be worth trying if anxiety and disorganization are significant problems.

In rarer situations, second-generation antipsychotic medications can also be used as a primary mood stabilizer for people who have not responded to other mood stabilizers. Clozapine, in particular, despite all of its risks and side effects, can be effective even when other mood stabilizers have not helped.

Choosing a Specific Antipsychotic Medication

All of the antipsychotic medications can be helpful in people with borderline disorder. Each has advantages and disadvantages, and it is often worth trying a second or third if the first does not work as hoped.

- *Risperidone (Risperidone)* is well tolerated when used at the 0.5–2 mg dose range often prescribed for people with a borderline disorder. It seems calming without being very sedating. However, even at this dose, risperidone can cause motor restlessness and prolactin elevation. It is available as an inexpensive generic medication, and seems to have the same mood stabilization and antidepressant effects as do all of the second-generation medications.
- *Quetiapine (Seroquel)* is the antipsychotic least likely to cause extrapyramidal side effects and most commonly used in people with borderline disorder, probably because of its sedation, which is generally considered desirable in this patient population (the sedation often helps a person sleep, and it decreases anxiety). Quetiapine is generally very well toler-

ated. It is often used over a wide dose range, from 25 mg up to several hundred mg a day. It can cause some weight gain, and the sedation that is helpful for one person can be a problem for another.

• *Aripiprazole (Abilify)* is mildly energizing for most people, rather than sedating, as are most antipsychotic medications. It is effective as an antipsychotic, as a mood stabilizer, and as a medication that can increase the effectiveness of antidepressant in people who have treatment resistant depression. There is some controlled research supporting its efficacy in people with borderline disorder. It generally is well tolerated with few side effects, and causes minimal weight gain. It can cause agitation and sleep problems, however, which can be significant for some people, and it can cause motor restlessness (akathisia) probably more often than the other second-generation antipsychotic medications. The most effective way to avoid this side effect is to start with a low dose, 2–5 mg, and increase over time as needed. The most effective way to treat akathisia, if it does occur, is to lower the dose. Aripiprazole is a long-acting medication with a half-life of around 70 hours, which means it can be taken any time during the day.

• *Ziprasidone (Geodon)* is a weight-neutral medication that is energizing for most people, rather than sedating, as are most antipsychotics. It sometimes causes agitation and sleep problems, however, which can become significant problems for some people. The agitation sometimes associated with ziprasidone can be treated with a benzodiazepine, which can present its own problem (dependence and abuse potential; see next section). Ziprasidone must be taken with food to be absorbed. A recent study failed to demonstrate that ziprasidone was effective for people with borderline disorder, but it is unclear if the problem was with the study or the medication. With ziprasidone, more is better. It is generally a more effective medication when used at 120 or 160 mg/day, then when used at a lower dose.

• *Olanzapine* is very effective, mildly sedating and generally well tolerated. Extrapyramidal side effects (EPS) are rarely a problem unless the does is raised above the level needed by most people diagnosed with borderline disorder. The biggest problem with olanzapine is the risk of weight gain, diabetes, and increased cholesterol. These do not occur in everyone, but do occur commonly and the weight gain can be very significant.

- *Clozapine* has more side effects and more risk than any of the other antipsychotic medications. There is good data that it can be more effective than other medications in people with schizophrenia, but there is no comparable data for any other group. In very rare situations, it may be worth trying clozapine as a mood stabilizer when no other medications have been effective.

(See Chapter 4 for more information about specific antipsychotic medications.)

Benzodiazepines

Addictive medications should be used rarely and with significant caution in people who have a history of other addictions. Given the high rate of substance abuse among people with borderline disorder and their tendency toward extremes, including impulsiveness, benzodiazepines should be used only rarely and cautiously in this population. Too often, attempts to use benzodiazepines to treat the anxiety that frequently accompanies borderline personality disorder end up further destabilizing the person. In particular, benzodiazepines should almost never be used in people who are already abusing alcohol or other drugs, no matter how much they request them or complain of anxiety.

If benzodiazepines are going to be used, there should be very clear target symptoms, and the amount of medication prescribed should be carefully monitored. If the person's behavior becomes more out of control, the benzodiazepines should be stopped immediately.

Medications for Symptoms Associated with PTSD

Many people with borderline disorder also meet diagnostic criteria for chronic PTSD. Although no medication is dramatically effective, the medications listed in Chapter 8, including prazosin, guanfacine, and clonidine, and can be very helpful in some people. (See Chapter 8 for more information.)

Omega-3 Fatty Acids

There are some data that a gram a day of omega-3 fatty acids can help both aggressive and depressive symptoms associated with borderline disorder. In one study, 1 gram a day of an omega-3 fatty acid was more effective than alprazolam.

Medication List
by Generic Name

Generic Name	Brand Name	Chief Action
acamprosate	Campral	anti-alcohol
alprazolam	Xanax	benzodiazepine/ antianxiety
amitriptyline	Elavil	tricyclic antidepressant
amoxapine	Ascendin	tricyclic antidepressant
amphetamine/ dextroamphetamine	Adderall	ADHD/stimulant
amphetamine/ dextroamphetamine	Adderall XR	ADHD/stimulant
aripiprazole	Abilify	Antipsychotic: second generation
aripiprazole fast dissolve	Abilify disc-melt	antipsychotic: second generation
atomoxetine	Strattera	ADHD: not a stimulant
benztropine	Cogentin	Antiparkinson medication
biperiden	Akineton	Antiparkinson medication
buprenorphine	Subutex	anti-opiate
buprenorphine/naloxone	Suboxone	anti-opiate
bupropion/Budeprion	Wellbutrin	antidepressant
buspirone	Buspar	antianxiety
carbamazepine	Carbatrol	mood stabilizer
carbamazepine	Tegretol	mood stabilizer
chlordiazepoxide	Librium	benzodiazepine/ antianxiety

Generic Name	Brand Name	Chief Action
chlorpromazine	Thorazine	antipsychotic: first generation
citalopram	Celexa	SSRI/SNRI antidepressant
clomipramine	Anafranil	tricyclic antidepressant used for OCD
clonazepam	Klonopin	benzodiazepine/ antianxiety
clonidine	Catapres	PTSD
clorazepate	Tranxene	benzodiazepine/ antianxiety
clozapine	Clozaril	antipsychotic: second generation
clozapine	FazaClo	antipsychotic: second generation
desipramine	Norpramin	tricyclic antidepressant
dexmethylphenidate	Focalin	ADHD/stimulant
diazepam	Valium	benzodiazepine/ antianxiety
diphenhydramine	Benadryl	Antiparkinson medication
disulfiram	Antabuse	anti-alcohol
divalproex sodium	Depakote	mood stabilizer
donepezil	Aricept	Alzheimer's medication
doxepin	Sinequan	tricyclic antidepressant
duloxetine	Cymbalta	SSRI/SNRI antidepressant
escitalopram	Lexapro	SSRI/SNRI antidepressant
estazolam	Prosom	benzodiazepine/ hypnotic
eszopiclone	Lunesta	sleeping pill
fluoxetine	Prozac	SSRI/SNRI antidepressant
fluphenazine	Prolixin	antipsychotic: first generation

Generic Name	Brand Name	Chief Action
fluphenazine long-acting injection	Prolixin decanoate	antipsychotic: first generation
flurazepam	Dalmane	benzodiazepine/ hypnotic
fluvoxamine	Luvox	SSRI/SNRI antidepressant
gabapentin	Neurontin	neurogenic pain/ fibromyalgia
galantamine	Razadyne	Alzheimer's medication
guanfacine	Tenex	PTSD
haloperidol	Haldol	antipsychotic: first generation
haloperidol long	Haldol decanoate	antipsychotic: first acting injection generation
hydroxyzine	Vistaril	sedating antihistamine
imipramine	Tofranil	tricyclic antidepressant
isocarboxazid	Marplan	MAOI antidepressant
L-methylfolate	Deplin	active metabolite of folic acid
lamotrigine	Lamictal	antidepressant/mood stabilizer
levothyroxine	Synthroid	thyroid hormone: T4
liothyronine	Cytomel	thyroid hormone: T3
lisdexamfetamine	Vyvanse	ADHD/stimulant
lithium	Eskalith	mood stabilizer
lorazepam	Ativan	benzodiazepine/ antianxiety
loxitane	Loxapine	antipsychotic: unusual first generation
maprotiline	Ludiomil	antidepressant
memantine	Namenda	Alzheimer's medication
methylphenidate	Concerta	ADHD/stimulant
methylphenidate	Metadate	ADHD/stimulant
methylphenidate	Ritalin	ADHD/stimulant
methylphenidate patch	Daytrana	ADHD/stimulant
modafanil	Provigil	stimulant
molindone	Moban	antipsychotic: unusual first generation
naltrexone	ReVia	anti-alcohol

Generic Name	Brand Name	Chief Action
naltrexone	Vivitrol	alcohol dependence
nefazodone	Serzone	antidepressant
nortriptyline	Pamelor	tricyclic antidepressant
olanzapine	Zyprexa	antipsychotic: second generation
olanzapine fast dissolve tablets	Zyprexa Zydis	antipsychotic: second generation
oxcarbazepine	Trileptal	mood stabilizer
paroxetine	Paxil	SSRI/SNRI antidepressant
perphenazine	Trilifon	antipsychotic: first generation
phenelzine	Nardil	MAOI antidepressant
pimozide	Orap	antipsychotic: first generation
pramipexole	Mirapex	restless legs syndrome
prazosin	Minipress	PTSD
pregabalin	Lyrica	neurogenic pain/ fibromyalgia
protriptyline	Vivactil	tricyclic antidepressant
quetiapine	Seroquel	antipsychotic: second generation
quetiapine long-acting	Seroquel XR	antipsychotic: second generation
ramelteon	Rozerem	sleeping pill
risperidone fast dissolve tablets	Risperdal m-tabs	antipsychotic: second generation
risperidone	Risperdal	antipsychotic: second generation
risperidone long-acting injection	Risperdal Consta	antipsychotic: second generation
rivastigmine	Exelon	Alzheimer's medication
ropinirole	Requip	restless legs syndrome
selegiline patch	Emsam	MAOI antidepressant
sertraline	Zoloft	SSRI/SNRI antidepressant
sodium oxybate	Xyrem	fibromyalgia
temazepam	Restoril	benzodiazepine/ hypnotic
thioridazine	Mellaril	antipsychotic: first generation

Generic Name	Brand Name	Chief Action
thiothixene	Navane	antipsychotic: first generation
topiramate	Topamax	alcohol dependence
tranylcypromine	Parnate	MAOI antidepressant
trazodone	Desyrel	sedating antidepressant used for sleep
triazolam	Halcion	benzodiazepine/ hypnotic
trifluoperazine	Stelazine	antipsychotic: first generation
trihexphenidyl	Artane	Antiparkinson medication
trimipramine	Surmontil	tricyclic antidepressant
varenicline	Chantix	smoking cessation
venlafaxine	Effexor	SSRI/SNRI antidepressant
zaleplon	Sonata	sleeping pill
ziprasidone	Geodon	antipsychotic: second generation
zolpidem	Ambien	sleeping pill
	D-cycloserine	augments behavioral therapy

Medication List
by Brand Name

Brand Name	Generic Name	Chief Action
Abilify	aripiprazole	Antipsychotic: second generation
Abilify disc-melt	aripiprazole fast dissolve	antipsychotic: second generation
Adderall	amphetamine/ dextroamphetamine	ADHD/stimulant
Adderall XR	amphetamine/ dextroamphetamine	ADHD/stimulant
Akineton	biperiden	Antiparkinson medication
Ambien	zolpidem	sleeping pill
Anafranil	clomipramine	tricyclic antidepressant used for OCD
Antabuse	disulfiram	anti-alcohol
Aricept	donepezil	Alzheimer's medication
Artane	trihexphenidyl	Antiparkinson medication
Ascendin	amoxapine	tricyclic antidepressant
Ativan	lorazepam	benzodiazepine/ antianxiety
Benadryl	diphenhydramine	Antiparkinson medication
Buspar	buspirone	antianxiety
Campral	acamprosate	anti-alcohol
Carbatrol	carbamazepine	mood stabilizer
Catapres	clonidine	PTSD
Celexa	citalopram	SSRI/SNRI antidepressant

Brand Name	Generic Name	Chief Action
Chantix	varenicline	smoking cessation
Clozaril	clozapine	antipsychotic: second generation
Cogentin	benztropine	Antiparkinson medication
Concerta	methylphenidate	ADHD/stimulant
Cymbalta	duloxetine	SSRI/SNRI antidepressant
D-cycloserine		augments behavioral therapy
Dalmane	flurazepam	benzodiazepine/ hypnotic
Daytrana	methylphenidate patch	ADHD/stimulant
Depakote	divalproex sodium	mood stabilizer
Deplin	L-methylfolate	active metabolite of folic acid
Desyrel	trazodone	sedating antidepressant used for sleep
Effexor	venlafaxine	SSRI/SNRI antidepressant
Elavil	amitriptyline	tricyclic antidepressant
Emsam	selegiline patch	MAOI antidepressant
Eskalith	lithium	mood stabilizer
Exelon	rivastigmine	Alzheimer's medication
FazaClo	clozapine	antipsychotic: second generation
Focalin	dexmethylphenidate	ADHD/stimulant
Geodon	ziprasidone	antipsychotic: second generation
Halcion	triazolam	benzodiazepine/ hypnotic
Haldol	haloperidol	antipsychotic: first generation
Haldol decanoate	haloperidol long acting injection	antipsychotic: first generation
Klonopin	clonazepam	benzodiazepine/ antianxiety
Lamictal	lamotrigine	antidepressant/mood stabilizer
Synthroid	levothyroxine	thyroid hormone: T4
Lexapro	escitalopram	SSRI/SNRI antidepressant

Brand Name	Generic Name	Chief Action
Librium	chlordiazepoxide	benzodiazepine/ antianxiety
Cytomel	liothyronine	thyroid hormone: T3
Loxapine	loxitane	antipsychotic: unusual first generation
Ludiomil	maprotiline	antidepressant
Lunesta	eszopiclone	sleeping pill
Luvox	fluvoxamine	SSRI/SNRI antidepressant
Lyrica	pregabalin	neurogenic pain/ fibromyalgia
Marplan	isocarboxazid	MAOI antidepressant
Mellaril	thioridazine	antipsychotic: first generation
Metadate	methylphenidate	ADHD/stimulant
Minipress	prazosin	PTSD
Mirapex	pramipexole	restless legs syndrome
Moban	molindone	antipsychotic: unusual first generation
Namenda	memantine	Alzheimer's medication
Nardil	phenelzine	MAOI antidepressant
Navane	thiothixene	antipsychotic: first generation
Neurontin	gabapentin	neurogenic pain/ fibromyalgia
Norpramin	desipramine	tricyclic antidepressant
Orap	pimozide	antipsychotic: first generation
Pamelor	nortriptyline	tricyclic antidepressant
Parnate	tranylcypromine	MAOI antidepressant
Paxil	paroxetine	SSRI/SNRI antidepressant
Prolixin	fluphenazine	antipsychotic: first generation
Prolixin decanoate	fluphenazine long-acting injection	antipsychotic: first generation
Prosom	estazolam	benzodiazepine/ hypnotic
Provigil	modafinil	stimulant
Prozac	fluoxetine	SSRI/SNRI antidepressant

Brand Name	Generic Name	Chief Action
Razadyne	galantamine	Alzheimer's medication
Requip	ropinirole	restless legs syndrome
Risperdal	risperidone	antipsychotic: second generation
Restoril	temazepam	benzodiazepine/ hypnotic
ReVia	naltrexone	anti-alcohol
Risperdal Consta	risperidone long-acting injection	antipsychotic: second generation
Risperdal m-tabs	risperidone fast dissolve tablets	antipsychotic: second generation
Ritalin	methylphenidate	ADHD/stimulant
Rozerem	ramelteon	sleeping pill
Seroquel	quetiapine	antipsychotic: second generation
Seroquel XR	quetiapine long-acting	antipsychotic: second generation
Serzone	nefazodone	antidepressant
Sinequan	doxepin	tricyclic antidepressant
Sonata	zaleplon	sleeping pill
Stelazine	trifluoperazine	antipsychotic: first generation
Strattera	atomoxetine	ADHD: not a stimulant
Suboxone	buprenorphine/naloxone	anti-opiate
Subutex	buprenorphine	anti-opiate
Surmontil	trimipramine	tricyclic antidepressant
Tegretol	carbamazepine	mood stabilizer
Tenex	guanfacine	PTSD
Thorazine	chlorpromazine	antipsychotic: first generation
Tofranil	imipramine	tricyclic antidepressant
Topamax	topiramate	alcohol dependence
Tranxene	clorazepate	benzodiazepine/ antianxiety
Trilifon	perphenazine	antipsychotic: first generation
Trileptal	oxcarbazepine	mood stabilizer
Valium	diazepam	benzodiazepine/ antianxiety
Vistaril	hydroxyzine	sedating antihistamine
Vivactil	protriptyline	tricyclic antidepressant

Brand Name	Generic Name	Chief Action
Vivitrol	naltrexone	alcohol dependence
Vyvanse	lisdexamfetamine	ADHD/stimulant
Wellbutrin	bupropion/Budeprion	antidepressant
Xanax	alprazolam	benzodiazepine/ antianxiety
Xyrem	sodium oxybate	fibromyalgia
Zoloft	sertraline	SSRI/SNRI antidepressant
Zyprexa	olanzapine	antipsychotic: second generation
Zyprexa Zydis	olanzapine fast dissolve tablets	antipsychotic: second generation

Medication List by Class

Antipsychotic Medications

chlorpromazine	Thorazine
fluphenazine	Prolixin
fluphenazine long-acting injection	Prolixin decanoate
haloperidol	Haldol
haloperidol long acting injection	Haldol decanoate
perphenazine	Trilifon
pimozide	Orap
thioridazine	Mellaril
thiothixene	Navane
trifluoperazine	Stelazine
aripiprazole	Abilify
aripiprazole fast dissolve	Abilify Discmelt
clozapine	Clozaril
clozapine	FazaClo
olanzapine	Zyprexa
olanzapine fast dissolve tablets	Zyprexa Zydis
quetiapine	Seroquel
risperidone	Risperdal
risperidone fast dissolve tablets	Risperdal m-tabs
risperidone long-acting injection	Risperdal Consta
quetiapine long-acting	Seroquel XR
ziprasidone	Geodon
loxitane	Loxapine
molindone	Moban

Antidepressant Medications

amitriptyline	Elavil
amoxapine	Ascendin
bupropion/Budeprion	Wellbutrin
citalopram	Celexa
clomipramine	Anafranil

desipramine	Norpramin
doxepin	Sinequan
duloxetine	Cymbalta
escitalopram	Lexapro
fluoxetine	Prozac
fluvoxamine	Luvox
imipramine	Tofranil
isocarboxazid	Marplan
maprotiline	Ludiomil
nefazodone	Serzone
nortriptyline	Pamelor
paroxetine	Paxil
phenelzine	Nardil
protriptyline	Vivactil
selegiline patch	Emsam
sertraline	Zoloft
tranylcypromine	Parnate
trimipramine	Surmontil
venlafaxine	Effexor

Mood Stabilizing Medications

carbamazepine	Carbatrol
carbamazepine	Tegretol
divalproex sodium	Depakote
lamotrigine	Lamictal
lithium	Eskalith
oxcarbazepine	Trileptal

Antianxiety Medications

alprazolam	Xanax
buspirone	Buspar
chlordiazepoxide	Librium
clonazepam	Klonopin
clorazepate	Tranxene
diazepam	Valium
lorazepam	Ativan

Sleeping Medications

estazolam	Prosom
eszopiclone	Lunesta
flurazepam	Dalmane
ramelteon	Rozerem
temazepam	Restoril
trazodone	Desyrel
triazolam	Halcion

| zaleplon | Sonata |
| zolpidem | Ambien |

Medications Used in the Treatment of Substance Abuse

acamprosate	Campral
buprenorphine	Subutex
buprenorphine/naloxone	Suboxone
disulfiram	Antabuse
naltrexone	ReVia
naltrexone	Vivitrol
topiramate	Topamax
varenicline	Chantix

Medications for PTSD

clonidine	Catapres
guanfacine	Tenex
prazosin	Minipress

Medications for Alzheimer's Disease

donepezil	Aricept
galantamine	Razadyne
memantine	Namenda
rivastigmine	Exelon

Miscellaneous Medications Discussed in the Book

benztropine	Cogentin
biperiden	Akineton
Cytomel	Liothyronine
diphenhydramine	Benadryl
gabapentin	Neurontin
hydroxyzine	Vistaril
L-methylfolate	Deplin
modafinil	Provigil
pramipexole	Mirapex
pregabalin	Lyrica
ropinirole	Requip
sodium oxybate	Xyrem
Synthroid	Levothyroxine
trihexphenidyl	Artane
d-cycloserine	

Medication List by Cost

Name	typical daily dose	generic cost × 30 days	Brand cost × 30 days
Antipsychotic Medications			
aripiprazole (Abilify)	15 mg/day	$376	
clozapine (Clozaril)	100 mg × 4/day	$201	
olanzapine (Zyprexa)	15 mg/day	$587	
paliperidone (Invega)	6 mg/day	$354	
quitiapine (Seroquel)	300 mg × 2/day	$602	
risperidone (Risperdal)	4 mg/day	$331	**$200
ziprasidone (Geodon)	80 mg × 2/day	$435	
halperidol (Haldol)	10 mg/day		$45
perphenazine (Trilifon)	16 mg/day		$28
Antidepressant Medications			
bupropion XL	300 mg/day	$220	$130
citalopram (Celexa)	40 mg/day	$104	$4
duloxetine (Cymbalta)	60 mg/day	$132	
escitalopram (Lexapro)	10 mg/day	$86	
fluoxetine (Prozac)	20 mg/day	$151	$4

mirtazapine (Remeron)	30 mg/day	$110	$27
venlafaxine XR	75 mg 3/day	$323	$102**
zoloft (Sertraline)	100 mg × 2/day	$104	$16

Mood Stabilizing Medication

lithium carbonate	300 mg × 4/day		$12
divalproex sodium	500 mg × 4/day	$392	$61
lamotrigine (Lamictal)	200 mg/day	$192	162**

Sleeping Pills

zolpidem (Ambien)	10 mg/day	$136	$18
zolpidem CR (Ambien CR)	12.5 mg/day	$126	
eszopiclone (Lunesta)	2mg /day	$169	

** These medications have very recently or are about to be available as an inexpensive generic, and the price is expected to drop precipitously early in 2010.

Significant cost savings can be achieved by "pill-splitting" some medications. For example, aripiprazole 15 mg # 30 is $378, 1/2 of a 30 mg tab costs $281. Escitalopram 10 mg × 30 is $86, 1/2 of a 20 mg tab costs $49.

Data from drugstore.com, with help from Scott Procknow of Genoa pharmacy.

Bibliography

PSYCHOPHARMACOLOGY BOOKS FOR NONPHYSICIANS

Dziegielewski, S.F. (2006). *Psychopharmacology handbook for the non-medically trained*. New York: Norton.

This book covers much of the same material as *Instant Psychopharmacology*, but it is written by a nonphysician and has a very different style. It has more general information about treatment, and less information about specific medications. It is another useful resource for the nonphysician looking for information in this general area.

Gitlin, M. J. (2007). *Psychotherapist's guide to psychopharmacology*. New York: Free Press.

Weiden, P. J., Scheifler, P. L., Diamond, R. J., & Ross, R. (1999). *Switching antipsychotic medications: A guide for consumers and families*. Arlington, VA: National Alliance for the Mentally Ill.

This guide provides basic information on the newer second-generation antipsychotic medications, with an emphasis on how to start one and how to switch from a traditional antipsychotic to one of the new medications. It includeds general information about how to most effectively use medications, as well as technical information about each of the second-generation antipsychotics. It is now a decade old, but still includes most of the medications in current use.

Witkovsky, M. T. (2009). *Instant psychpharmacology for children and adolescents*. New York: Norton.

My book does not cover any mention of children; this gap is filled by Michael Witkovsky's new book. Children are not just small adults.

Treatment of children is a specialized area, and both assessment and treatment are very different in children than in adults. Information about the treatment of kids needs to come from someone with a focus in this area, someone who is a child psychiatrist like the author of this book.

GENERAL PSYCHOPHARMACOLOGY TEXTS

Janicak, P. G., David, J. M., Preskorn, S. H., Ayd, F. J., Marder, S. R., & Pavuluri, M. N. (2006). *Principles and practice of psychopharmacology (4th ed.)*. Philadelphia: Lippincott, Williams & Wilkins.
This is a more definitive textbook, better referenced with more of the research support for statements. It is written by a group of the most distinguished psychopharmacologists in the country. It is an excellent reference book.

Lieberman, J. A., & Tasman, A. (2006). *Handbook of psychiatric drugs*. New York: Wiley.
A brief handbook that has essential facts with little elaboration and little description of mechanism. Lists relevant indications and side effects.

Perry, P. J., Alexander, B., Liskow B. I., & DeVane, C. L. (2007). *Psychotropic drug handbook (8th ed.)* Philadelphia: Lippincott, Williams & Wilkins.
A very good book, up to date and complete. This is more than a handbook, but less than a fully referenced textbook. This (or the Schatzberg manual, below) would be a very good choice for a general psychopharmacology book.

Schatzberg, A. F., Cole, J. O., & DeBattista, C. (2007). *Manual of clinical psychopharmacology (6th ed.)*. Washington, DC: American Psychiatric Press.
A very good book, up to date and complete. This is more than a handbook, but less than a fully referenced textbook. This (or the Perry manual, above) would be a very good choice for a general psychopharmacology book.

Schatzberg, A. F., & Nemeroff, C. B. (2009). *Textbook of psychopharmacology* (4th ed.). Washington, DC: American Psychiatric Press.

Previous editions of this book have been one of the definitive reference works in psychopharmacology.

SPECIALIZED REFERENCE BOOKS

Bezchlibnyk-Butler, K. Z., & Jeffries, J. J. (2007). *Clinical handbook of psychotropic drugs (17th ed.)*. Kirkland, WA: Hogrefe & Huber.
This book is a compendium of lists and tables. It is the definitive reference for looking up specific data of information about individual medications and classes of medication.

Drug facts and comparisons 2009. St. Louis, MI: Walters Kluwer Health.
This book is a compendium of all prescribed medications with indications and side effects, including very useful summary tables. It covers the same material as the *PDR*, but is much more readable. Unfortunately, it is also much more expensive than the *PDR*. There is a pocket version that is much less expensive and covers basic information.

Physicians' desk reference (PDR) (63rd ed.). (2009). Des Moines, IO: Medical Economics.
This book lists every prescription medication marketed in the United States, along with indications, approved dose ranges, and side effects. It has indexes for medications by trade name, by generic name, and by drug category. Unfortunately, it is difficult to interpret information in this book. For example, it lists every reported side effect without giving information about which side effects are common and which have only been reported once, which are serious and which are trivial. *Drug Facts and Comparisons* covers similar information in a more user-friendly format (see above), but the *PDR* is more readily available.

Stahl, S. M. (2008). *Essential psychopharmacology: Neuroscientific basis and practical applications (3rd ed.)*. New York: Cambridge University Press.
This is an excellent, very readable book on neurotransmitters, receptors, and the basic science of how medications work.

It is not useful as a clinical guide, but is highly recommended for someone who wants a more theoretical understanding of psychopharmacology.

Julien, R. M. (2007). *A primer of drug action (11th ed.)*. New York: Worth Publishers.
This is an excellent, very readable overview of how medications work, how the brain is organized, and how receptors work. It includes a very useful section on the mechanism of drugs of abuse, including marijuana, hallucinogens, and anabolic steroids. It is somewhat technical and is not useful as a clinical guide, but is highly recommended for a more theoretical understanding of drug action.

USEFUL BOOKS, EVEN IF NOT ABOUT PSYCHOPHARMACOLOGY

American Psychiatric Association. (2000). *Diagnostic and statistical manual of mental disorders, fourth edition, text revision (DSM-IV-TR)*. Washington, DC: Author.
This is the current diagnostic manual being used in the United States. There is also a smaller *Quick Reference Guide* available, which includes all of the diagnoses and definitions, but does not include the background material.

Diamond, R. J. and Scheifler, P. L. (2007). *Treatment collaboration: Improving the therapist, prescriber, client relationship*. New York: Norton.
Prescribers decide what medications to prescribe for a client, who is often much better known by a therapist or case manager, and the client will then decide whether to really take it. The issue of the relationship between the prescriber, therapist, and consumer is a critical part of all effective treatment, including effective use of medication. This is a practical book about how to work with the complexities of these relationships.

Fadiman, A. (1997). *The spirit catches you and you fall down*. New York: Farrar, Straus & Giroux.
This book has nothing to do with psychopharmacology, but it

is required reading for all medical students who take an elective with me. On the surface it is about the conflict between a very well meaning set of physicians, and a very loving Hmong family dealing with a daughter with severe epilepsy. It is really about how our own values and beliefs color everything we do. If you are part of a struggle over whether medication is really needed or whether someone really has a mental illness, then you too should read this book. It isone of the more important books that I have read over the past several years.

Linehan, M. M. (1993). *Cognitive–behavioral treatment of borderline personality disorder*. New York: Guilford Press.

This continues to be the definitive book in the treatment of people with this diagnosis. It is practical, thoughtful, and respectful of the struggles that people are experiencing.

Miller, W. R., & Rollnick, S. (2001). *Motivational interviewing (2nd ed.)*. New York: Guilford Press.

This is the most important book that I have read in several years. It is required reading for students who work with me. Although it is written with a focus on drug and alcohol treatment, it is entirely relevant to rethinking how to help people change their own behavior.

SELF-HELP BOOKS

There are a large number of excellent self-help books now available. The best of them teach about the underlying disorder and then take a practical, behavioral, or cognitive–behavioral approach to treatment. Many of these approaches are based on controlled research. Those listed below are those on my bookshelf. Many others are equally good. I think that self-help books are underused by most clinicians.

ADHD

Safren, S. A., Sprich, S., Perlman, C. A., & Otto, M. W. (2005). Mastering your adult ADHD: A cognitive–behavioral treatment program. New York: Oxford University Press.

Anxiety Disorders

Barlow, D. H., & Craske, M. G. (2000). *Mastery of your anxiety and panic: Therapist guide (4th ed.).* New York: Oxford University Press.
This is one of the standard self-help books that we give to people who come into our clinic with complaints of anxiety and panic. It is practical and very user friendly.

Beckfield, D. F. (2003). *Master your panic and take back your life (3rd ed.).* Atascadero, CA: Impact Publishers.
This is an excellent, practical, and highly readable self-help book for dealing with panic disorder.

Craske, M. G. & Barlow, D. H. Mastery of your anxiety and worry. New York: Oxford University Press.

Bourne, E. J. (2005). *The anxiety and phobia workbook (4th ed.).* Oakland, CA: New Harbinger.

Hyman, B. M. & Pedrick, C. (2005). *The OCD workbook (2nd ed.).* Your guide to breaking free from obsessive–conmpulsive disorder. Oakland, CA: New Harbinger Publications.

Penzel, F. (2003). *The hair-pulling problem: A complete guide to trichotillomania.* New York: Oxford University Press.

Purdon, C. & Clark, D. A. (2005). *Overcoming obsessive thoughts.* Oakland, CA: New Harbinger Publications.

Bipolar Disorder

Basco, M. R. *The bipolar workbook: Tools for controlling your mood swings.* New York: Guilford Press.

Borderline Disorder

Linehan, M. M. (1993). *Skills training manual for treating borderline pesonality disorder.* New York: Guilford Press.

Depression

Burns, D. D. (1999). *Feeling good: The new mood therapy (rev. ed.).* Harper.

Greenberger, D., & Padesky, C. A. (1995). *Mind over mood*. New York: Guilford Press.

This is a self-help and clinician training manual for dealing with depression. It is based on the principles of cognitive–behavioral therapy initially developed by Aaron Beck. There are many self-help books for depression, and there may be others that are as good as this one. This is the one that I know and use. I regularly suggest that almost all of the clients that I see with depression read this book, along with their families.

Insomnia

Hauri, P., Jarman, M., & Linde, S. (2001). *No more sleepless nights*. New York: Wiley.

This book, along with its companion workbook, are excellent self-help tools for people with insomnia.

Crisis Intervention

Copeland, M. E. (1997). *Wellness recovery action plan: WRAP*. West Dummerston, VT: Peach Press.

WRAP is an effective way to help consumers stay in control of their own life. Whether one wishes to use a formal WRAP or a more simplified version, this book is a must-read for anyone working with consumers who are at risk for going into crisis, and for consumers who may find themselves in crisis.

RECENT REVIEW ARTICLES ON MEDICATION AND BORDERLINE PERSONALITY DISORDER

Abraham, P. F., Calabrese, J. R. Evidence-based pharmacologic treatment of borderline personality disorder: A shift from SSRIs to anticonvulsants and atypical antipsychotics? *J Affect Disord* 2008 Nov;111(1):21–30.

Medications for borderline personality disorder. *Carlat Psychiatric Report* 2008 Sept; 3–8.

NEWSLETTERS

These are a number of psychopharmacology newsletters that survey the literature and provide very short practical and up-to-date overviews of current research. They are easy ways to stay informed about the latest developments. They are all a bit different, and all are excellent. They are designed for physicians and other people who are already knowledgable about psychopharmacology. The four that I read are:

The Carlatt Psychiatry Report (www.thecarlatreport.com)

This is my favorite newsletter, and the one that I read first when it arrives. It is unbiased, takes no money from pharmaceutical companies, and has a refreshingly iconoclastic style in its medication reviews. It tends to focus on a few medications every month and does not attempt to cover the recent literature as much as the other newsletters.

The following three newsletters all review the current literature, with relatively less editorial input. They are all fairly expensive, but are a fast way to review what is being published in current journals. There are a number of other similar newsletters that are probably as good, but that I do not personally read.

Biological Therapies in Psychiatry (www.btpnews.com)
Gelenberg, A. (Ed.). Published by Healthcare Technology Systems.

Psychiatry Drug Alerts (psych@alertpubs.com)
Journal Watch Psychiatry, published by Massachusetts Medical Society (http://psychiatry.jwatch.org/).

Brown University Psychopharmacology Update

(http://www3.interscience.wiley.com/journal/110575470/home) Price, L. (Ed.). Published by Wiley.

COMPUTER-BASED RESOURCES

Epocrates is a program for a Palm PDA that gives basic information about every medication in the PDR. It is free and can be downloaded from www.epocrates.com.

WEB SITES

Web sites to go for reliable, current information about medications:
http://www.drugsimple.com/
Drug Simple is a quick way to look up basic information about all prescription medications. It is not as complete a some of the other medication data bases, but it is free and easy to use.

http://www.nlm.nih.gov/medlineplus/druginformation.html
Medline Plus from the U.S. National Library of Medicine provides reliable information about all medications avialable in the United States, including herbs and supplements.
Web site for up-to-date information on drug–drug information:
http://medicine.iupui.edu/flockhart/table.htm
Flockhart, D. A. Drug Interactions: Cytochrome P450 Drug Interaction Table. Indiana University School of Medicine (2007).

Web site for information on herbal preparations, and interactions between herbal remedies and prescribed medications:
http://www.personalhealthzone.com/herbsafety.html

Web sites for a wide variety of information about mental health problems (some of these websites also include information about medications):

http://www.mentalhealth.com
A web page of general mental health information, including a pointer to a pharmacology page that includes basic information about almost every prescription medication available in the United States.

http://www.nami.org/
Web page for the National Alliance for the Mentally Ill. This is not really a page about psychopharmacology, but it is still a useful reference. Every professional, family member, and consumer who is dealing with serious mental illness should know about NAMI. If you do not know about them, visit their web page.

http://www.samhsa.gov/
The Substance Abuse and Mental Health Services Administration (SAMHSA) is a website with a lot of good general information about statistics, grants, and government initiatives, but not much about medications.

http://www.mentalhealth.org/
This is the knowledge exchange website of the Center for Mental Health Services. It includes links to many other websites and allows access to all of the Surgeon General's reports as well as to a searchable link "Mental Health Resources on the Internet."

Specialized site for information about dangerous or unusual medication side effects:

http://www.fda.gov/medwatch/
FDA medwatch: You can search for FDA warnings about medications easily via a simple search engine at the website. You can also go into the FDA web page to look at the data presented for new medication approvals, but this information is not well indexed and is often difficult to find.

www.womensmentalhealth.org
This web site provides up-to-date information on psychiatric disorders during pregnancy, and the use od medication while pregnant or breastfeeding.

Index

Abilify. *see* aripiprazole
absorption, 29
acamprosate, 234–35
acetylcholine, 25–26
   Alzheimer's disease and, 230
adrenergic system
   definition, 118
   down-regulation of, in PTSD
    treatment, 218–20
   see also epinephrine
agitation
   antipsychotic therapy, 52, 81
   benzodiazepine therapy, 193
   dementia-associated, 81
agonist medications, 25
agranulocytosis
   antipsychotic medication side
    effect, 75–76, 79
   monitoring for, 144
   mood-stabilizing medication
    side effect, 174
akathisia
   antipsychotic medication side
    effects, 64, 96
   assessment, 13–14
   beta-blocker therapy, 214–15
   complications, 63–64
   symptoms, 63
   treatment, 64, 192–93
akinesia, 64
alcohol dependence treatment,
   232, 233–36

alcohol withdrawal, 193
allergic reactions
   antidepressant medications,
    144
   prevention, 5
alpha-1 adrenergic receptor blockers, 23, 219–20
alpha-2 adrenergic agonists, 23,
   220
alpha-2 antagonists, 21
alpha-adrenergic side effects, 67
alpha-amino-3-hydroxy-5-methyl-
   4-isoxazole-propionic acid
   (AMPA), 28
alprazalom, 187–88, 195
Alzheimer's disease, 229–32, 269
amantadine, 212–13
Ambien. *see* zolpidem
amitryptyline, 205–6
AMPA. *see* alpha-amino-3-hydroxy-
   5-methyl-4-isoxazole-propi-
   onic acid
amphetamines, 221–23, 224–25,
   226*t*
Anafranil. *see* clomipramine
Anatabuse. *see* disulfiram
anger control, 160
anhedonia, 120–21
Antabuse. *see* disulfiram
antagonist medications, 25
antianxiety medications. *see* anxiolytic medications

anticholinergic drugs, 23
  abuse potential, 212
  dosage, 211
  indications, 210
  mechanism of action, 210–11,
    211
  pharmacology, 25–26
  side effects, 46, 66, 143, 211–12
anticholinesterase inhibitors, 229,
    230–31
anticonvulsant drugs, 22, 155
antidepressant medications
  as antianxiety medications,
    200
  assessment for treatment with,
    117–18
  augmentation, 150–51, 159–60,
    163, 215
  bipolar disorder and, 119–20
  borderline personality disorder
    treatment, 250–51
  classification, 19, 21–22,
    115–16, 125–26
  costs, 270–71
  depression treatment, 114–15,
    120–22
  failure, 116
  with indirect action on sero-
    tonin and norepinephrine,
    137–39
  with indirect dopaminergic
    action, 139–41
  list of, 267–68
  long-term use, 116–17
  mechanism of action, 118,
    125–26
  pegnancy and, 4–5
  side effects, 152*t*
  for sleeping problems, 137,
    204–6
  therapeutic applications, 115,
    120–25
  treatment decisions, 150–51
  types of, 2–3

withdrawal, 120
  see also selective serotonin
    reuptake inhibitors; serotonin
    and norepinephrine reuptake
    inhibitors; *specific medication*
antihistamines, 23, 207, 228
antiparkinsonian medications, 23,
    209–13
antipsychotic medications
  for acute mania of bipolar disor-
    der, 55–56
  for bipolar depression, 57–58
  borderline personality disorder
    treatment, 252–55
  classification, 20–21, 37, 101–2
  costs, 43, 270
  for delusional depression, 58
  for dementia and delirium,
    58–59
  discontinuing, 51–52
  dosing, 49–51
  drug–drug interactions, 59–60
  effectiveness, 44–45
  indications, 37, 38, 48–59
  injection medications, 42–43,
    106–9
  list of, 267
  mechanism of action, 26–27,
    38–42, 71
  newer drugs, 97–98
  for ongoing treatment of bipolar
    disorder, 56–57
  side effects, 45–48, 61–69, 100,
    101, 109–13
  side effect treatment, 209–13
  use during pregnancy, 69–70
  see also first-generation antipsy-
    chotic medications; second-
    generation antipsychotic
    medications
anxiety
  antidepressant medication
    therapy, 122–24, 200
  antipsychotic drug therapy, 89

beta-blocker therapy, 214
mood-stabilizing medications
for, 179, 180–81
see also anxiolytic medications
anxiolytic medications, 22
list of, 268
mechanism of action, 27
sleep-promoting medications
and, 185–86
specificity, 185
without sleep effects, 197–200
see also benzodiazepines
Aricept. *see* donepezil
aripiprazole
for acute mania of bipolar disorder, 56
advantages, 93, 94
borderline personality disorder
treatment, 254
indications, 94–95
mechanism of action, 93–94
side effects, 64, 95–96
Arkineton. *see* biperiden
Artane. *see* trihexphenidyl
asenapine, 97–98
assessment
allergy risk, 5
for antidepressant therapy,
117–18
for antipsychotic therapy, 48
attention-deficit/hyperactivity
disorder, 221
for borderline personality disorder treatment, 244–45
good practice, 4
before initiating treatment,
14–15
medication failure, 16–18
participants, 7
sleep problems, 191–92,
200–202
atenolol, 198–99, 216
Ativan. *see* lorazepam
atomoxetine, 136, 227–28

attention-deficit/hyperactivity
disorder, 23, 220–23, 226–27,
228–29
atypical antipsychotics. *see* second-
generation antipsychotic
medications
autism, 81

Benadryl. *see* diphenhydramine
benzodiazepines, 22–23
addictive potential, 187, 195
for akathisia, 192–93
borderline personality disorder
treatment, 255
differences among, 187–89
drug–drug interactions, 78–79
indications, 186, 190–93
mechanism of action, 186–87
muscle spasm treatment, 193
overdose, 186–87
for promoting sleep, 189, 191–92
to reduce agitation, 193
to reduce side effects of other
medications, 192–93
side effects, 196
for sleep problems, 202–3
to treat alcohol withdrawal, 193
use during pregnancy, 196–97
withdrawal, 195–96
see also diazepam; flurazepam;
lorazepam; temazepam
benztropine, 66, 211
beta-blockers, 23, 197, 198–99
atypical, 215
dosage and administration, 216
indications, 213, 214–15
mechanism of action, 27,
213–14
side effects, 216–17
biperiden, 211
bipolar disorder
acute mania treatment, 55–56
antidepressant medications and,
119–20

bipolar disorder (*continued*)
   antipsychotic drug therapy, 88,
      95, 156
   clinical characteristics, 157
   depression treatment, 57–58
   mood-stabilizing medications
      for, 156–57, 158–59, 167, 171,
      176, 177
   ongoing treatment, 56–57
birth defects. *see* pregnancy, medication use during
blood–brain barrier, 30
blood dyscrasia, 68
borderline personality disorder
   antidepressant therapy, 250–51
   antipsychotic therapy, 89,
      252–55
   clinical conceptualization, 239,
      240–41
   core deficits, 241–42
   mood-stabilizing medications
      for, 160, 247–50
   PTSD symptoms in, 255–56
   therapeutic assumptions, 243–44
   therapeutic relationship and,
      245
   treatment strategies and design,
      239–40, 242–43, 244–47
brand names, drug, 262–66
bulimia, 124
buphrenorphine, 236–37
bupropion, 125, 139–41, 237, 250
BuSpar. *see* buspirone
buspirone, 197–98
butyrophenomes, 21

calcium channel blockers, 183–84
Campral. *see* acamprosate
carbamazepine, 20
   borderline personality disorder
      treatment, 248
   dosage, 171–72
   drug-drug interactions, 32,
      170–71, 175
   indications, 155, 171
      laboratory monitoring, 172,
         174–75
      serum levels, 172
      side effects, 173–75
      use during pregnancy, 173
cardiovascular problems
   antidepressant medication side
      effects, 143
   antipsychotic medication side
      effects, 76, 91–93
   beta-blocker therapy for, 214
Catapres. *see* clonidine
Celexa. *see* citalopram
Chantix. *see* varenicline
chlordiazepoxide, 188, 194
chlorpromazine, 67, 69, 101, 102–3
cholinergic medications, 23
cholinergic receptors, 25
cimetidine, 175
citalopram, 128, 150
classes of medications, 2–3, 19,
   20–23, 267–69. *see also spe-*
   cific class
client considerations in pharmacotherapy, 9–12
clomipramine, 200
clonazepam, 187–88, 195
clonidine, 219
clozapine
   borderline personality disorder
      treatment, 255
   cost, 76–77
   dose, 77
   drug–drug interactions, 78–79,
      175
   effectiveness, 44–45
   generic formulations, 76
   indications, 72
   prescribing practice, 43, 77–78
   side effects, 43, 62, 66, 69, 71,
      72–76
Clozaril. *see* clozapine
Cogentin. *see* benztropine
cognitive–behavioral therapy,
   151–53

communicating with client, 7–8
communicating with physicians,
    8–9
compliance, 12–14
consultations, 5–6
contraceptives, 175
cost of medication, 34–36, 270–71
    antipsychotic medications, 43
    clozapine, 76–77
Cymbalta. *see* duloxetine
cytochrome P450 enzymes, 34, 134

Dalmane. *see* flurazepam
D-cycloserine, 197, 199–200
delirium, 14, 58–59
dementia, 58–59
Demerol. *see* meperidine
Depakene. *see* valproic acid
Depakote. *see* valproic acid
Deplin. *see* L-methyfolate   ´
depression
    antidepressant therapy, 114–15,
        120–22
    antipsychotic drug therapy,
        80–81, 85, 88, 95
    in bipolar disorder, 57–58
    classification, 121
    delusional, 58
    folic acid deficiency and, 149
    life stress and, 114
    mood-stabilizing medications
        for, 159–60, 163
    stimulant medications for,
        223–24
    treatment strategies, 114–15,
        150–54
    see also antidepressant medica-
        tions
desvenlafaxine, 132
Desyrel. *see* trazodone
Dexedrine. *see* amphetamine
dextroamphetamine, 224, 225
dextromethorphan, 147–48
diabetes, as antipsychotic drug side
    effect, 61–62, 73–74, 83

diazepam, 185, 188, 194
diphenhydramine, 66, 207, 212
disulfiram, 233
divalproex sodium, 78, 166–67,
    168, 248. *see also* valproic
    acid
donepezil, 231
dopaminergic drugs, 23
    antipsychotic medications,
        38–42, 209–10, 212
    mechanism of action, 24–25
    pharmacology, 26–27
dopaminergic system
    amphetamine action, 224
    antidepressants with indirect
        action on, 139–41
    dopamine pathways, 39–40
    dopamine receptors, 38–39
dosage
    cautions, 2
    evaluating medication failure,
        17
    initiating treatment, 15
doxepin, 205–6
drug-drug interactions
    current understanding, 31–34
    prevention, 4
    significance of, 3–4
    see also specific drug
duloxetine, 131–32
dysthymia, 121
dystonia, 63

Effexor. *see* venlafaxine
Elavil. *see* amitriptyline
electroconvulsive therapy, 151
Emsam. *see* selegiline patch
epinephrine, 27, 213
erythromycin, 78, 175
escitalopram, 128–29
Eskalith. *see* lithium
eszopiclone, 204
excitatory neurotransmitters, 24
Exelon. *see* rivastigmine
exercise, 153

extrapyramidal motor system,
  39–40, 62
extrapyramidal symptoms
  antipsychotic medication side
    effects, 46, 62–65
  source, 39–40
  treatment, 209–13
  types of, 46, 210

fibromyalgia, 125
  mood-stabilizing medications
    for, 179, 180
first-generation antipsychotic medi-
    cations, 20–21, 37
  effectiveness, 44–45
  injections, 107–8
  mechanism of action, 26
  potency classification, 101–2
  side effects, 45, 46, 101, 110–11
  technical development, 101
  see also antipsychotic medi-
    cations; chlorpromazine;
    fluphenazine; haloperidol;
    loxapine; perphenazine;
    thioridazine; thiothixene
fluoxetine
  antianxiety action, 200
  cost, 128
  dosage, 128
  drug–drug interactions, 3,
    32–33, 131, 134, 142, 148
fluphenazine, 104
fluphenazine decanoate, 107, 108
flurazepam, 185, 188, 202–3
fluvoxamine, 134
folic acid, 149, 169
Food and Drug Administration, 19
food–drug interactions, 146–47
frontal cortex, dopamine pathway,
  39

GABA. see gamma-aminobutyric
  acid
GABA-A agonists, 203–4
gabapentin

borderline personality disorder
  treatment, 249–50
dosage, 180
indications, 155, 179
side effects, 180
Gabitril. see tiagabine
galantamine, 231
gamma-aminobutyric acid (GABA),
  27, 186–87
generalized anxiety disorder,
  123–24
generic drugs, 5, 35, 257–61
Geodon. see ziprasidone
glutamate, 27–28, 229, 231
grapefruit juice, 33
guanfacine, 220

hair loss, valproic acid side effect,
  169
Halcion. see triazolam
Haldol. see haloperidol
half-life, 29–30
haloperidol, 53, 54, 103–4, 175
haloperidol decanoate, 107–8
heat stroke, antipsychotic side
  effect, 68–69, 74
heroin addiction treatment, 236–37
HIV medications, 135
5-HT. see serotonin
hydrochlorothiazide, 165, 166
hypnotics. see sleeping pills
hyponatremia, antidepressant side
  effect, 133

iloperidone, 97
impulsive behavior, 181–82
Inderal. see propranolol
indication, FDA, 19–20
informed consent, 7–8
inhibitory neurotransmitters, 24
injectable antipsychotic medica-
    tions, 42–43, 106–9
Invega. see paliperidone

Klonopin. see clonazepam

Lamictal. *see* lamotrigine
lamotrigine
   borderline personality disorder
    treatment, 249
   dosage, 178–79
   drug-drug interactions, 171, 175
   indications, 177
   side effects, 177–78, 179
Lexapro. *see* escitalopram
Librium. *see* chlordiazepoxide
limbic system dopamine pathway,
   39
lisdexamfetamine, 225
lithium
   dosage, 162–63
   drug-drug interactions, 166
   formulations, 158
   indications, 155, 158–60
   laboratory monitoring, 160–62,
    163
   long-term effects, 164–65
   overdose risk, 166
   side effects, 163–65
   use during pregnancy, 166
Lithobid. *see* lithium
L-methyfolate, 149–50
lorazepam, 54, 185, 194–95
loxapine, 105
Loxitane. *see* loxapine
Lunesta. *see* eszopiclone
Luvox. *see* fluvoxamine
Lyrica. *see* pregabalin

major depression, 121
mania
   antidepressant medication side
    effects, 119–20, 144
   antipsychotic drug therapy, 80,
    84, 155–56
   hypomania, 157–58
   see also bipolar disorder
marketing of medications, 35–36
melatonin, 206–7
Mellaril. *see* thioridazine
memantine, 232

memory impairment
   anticholinergic drug side effects,
    211
   benzodiazepine effects, 196
   topiramate effects, 182
meperidine, 147
mesocortical pathway, 39
mesolimbic pathway, 39, 41
metabolic acidosis, 236
metabolic syndrome, 83
methadone, 236
methamphetamine, 225
methylphenidate, 221–23, 226–27
Minipress. *see* prazosin
mirtazapine, 138–39, 200, 205, 250
Moban. *see* molindone
modafinil, 228
monoamine oxidase inhibitors, 22
   borderline personality disorder
    treatment, 250–51
   clinical applications, 145
   dosage, 145–46
   drug–drug interactions, 135,
    147–48
   food interactions, 146–47
   mechanism of action, 145, 146
   side effects, 148
   skin patch, 145, 147
   withdrawal, 148–49
monoamines, 118
mood-stabilizing medications, 22
   antipsychotic drugs as, 155–56
   borderline personality disorder
    treatment, 160, 247–50
   costs, 271
   indications, 155, 156–57
   list of, 268
   technical development, 155
   treatment decisions, 157
   see also carbamazepine; gaba-
    pentin; lamotrigine; lithium;
    oxcarbazepine; pregabalin;
    tiagabine; topiramate; valp-
    roic acid; verapamil
muscarinic receptors, 25–26

naloxone, 236–37
naltrexone, 233–34
Namenda. see memantine
narcolepsy, 224
Nardil. see phenelzine
Navane. see thiothixene
nefazodone, 138
neuroleptic malignant syndrome,
    68
neuroleptics. see first-generation
    antipsychotic medications
Neurontin. see gabapentin
neuropathic pain, 124–25
    mood-stabilizing medications
    for, 179, 180
neurotransmitters, 24–25, 127
nicotine replacement, 23
nicotinic receptors, 25–26
nigrostriatal pathway, 39
NMDA. see N-methyl-d-aspartate
NMDA agonists, 23, 199
NMDA antagonists, 229, 231–32
N-methyl-d-aspartate (NMDA), 28
norepinephrine, 28
    antidepressants with indirect
        action on, 137–39
    see also serotonin and norepi-
        nephrine reuptake inhibitors
norepinephrine and dopamine
    reuptake blockers, 21
norepinephrine antidepressants, 21
norepinephrine reuptake inhibitor,
    21, 227–28
Norpramin. see desipramine
nortriptyline, 3

obsessive–compulsive disorder,
    123, 129
    anxiolytic therapy, 197, 199–200
    benzodiazepine use and,
        190–91
olanzapine, 51, 109
    for acute mania of bipolar disor-
        der, 56
    advantages, 82

borderline personality disorder
    treatment, 254–55
    formulations, 82
    indications, 84–85
    side effects, 62, 67, 82–84
omega-3 fatty acids, 256
opiate dependence, 236–37
oxazepam, 188
oxcarbazepine
    advantages, 176
    borderline personality disorder
        treatment, 248
    dosage, 176
    indications, 176
    metabolization, 175–76
    side effects, 176–77

P450 enzyme system, 34, 134
paliperidone, 67, 96, 109
Palmitate. see paliperidone
pancreatitis, valproic acid side
    effect, 170
panic disorder, 122–23, 191
Parkinson's disease and Parkinson-
    like symptoms, 23, 63, 209–10
Parnate. see tranylcypromine
paroxetine, 33, 129, 134
partial agonists, 25, 197
Paxil. see paroxetine
performance anxiety, 198–99, 214
perphenazine, 104
personality disorders, 160
pharmaceutical industry, 19–20,
    35–36
phenelzine, 146. see also monoam-
    ine oxidase inhibitors
phenothiazines, 21
Physicians' Desk Reference, 2
pindolol, 215
polycystic ovaries, 170
posttraumatic stress disorder, 23,
    124
    beta-blocker therapy to prevent,
        215
    clinical features, 217–18

medication list, 269
symptoms in borderline personality disorder, 255–56
treatment, 218–20
prazosin, 219–20
pregabalin
   borderline personality disorder treatment, 250
   dosage, 181
   indications, 180–81
   side effects, 180, 181
pregnancy, medication use during
   antidepressant medications, 136
   antipsychotic medications, 69–70
   benzodiazepines, 196–97
   carbamazepine, 173
   cautions in prescribing, 4–5
   lithium, 166
   valproic acid, 168–69
prescribing practice
   assessment, 48
   client perspective, 9–12
   cost considerations, 34–36
   essential rules, 2–6
   FDA indications and, 19–20
   initiating treatment, 15–16
   before initiating treatment, 14–15
   medication failure, 16–18
   to promote compliance, 12–14
   resources, 2
   sleeping pills, 200–202
   therapeutic and professional relationships in, 6–8
   therapeutic goals, 9, 11, 15
   therapist's role, 1
   time considerations, 28–31
priapism, 137, 205
primary excitatory neurotransmitter, 27–28
primary inhibitory neurotransmitter, 27
Pristiq. *see* desvenlafaxine
prolactin, side effects of antipsychotic medications, 40, 67, 79, 82–83

Prolixin. *see* fluphenazine
propranolol, 198–99, 214–15, 216
Provigil. *see* modafanil
Prozac. *see* fluoxetine
pseudo-parkinsonianism, 63
psychosis, dementia-associated, 81
psychotherapy
   depression treatment, 114–15, 151–53
   substance abuse treatment, 232
psychotoxic side effects of antipsychotic medications, 66
PTSD. *see* posttraumatic stress disorder
pyramidal system, 39

quetiapine, 51, 53
   for acute mania of bipolar disorder, 55–56
   advantages, 85
   borderline personality disorder treatment, 253–54
   formulations, 85
   indications, 86–89
   mechanism of action, 85–86
   side effects, 67, 86

ramelteon, 206–7
rashes, 144, 174, 178
Razadyne. *see* galantamine
Remeron. *see* mirtazapine
Reminyl. *see* galantamine
research and development, 19–20
resistance to pharmacotherapy, 9–10
Restoril. *see* temazepam
ReVia. *see* naltrexone
Risperal. *see* risperidone
risperidone, 43, 50–51
   for acute mania of bipolar disorder, 56
   borderline personality disorder treatment, 253
   cost, 82

risperidone (continued)
    drug-drug interactions, 33
    formulations, 79
    indications, 79-81
    microspheres, 108-9
    side effects, 64, 67, 79
Ritalin. see methylphenidate
rivastigmine, 231
roboxetine. see atomoxetine
Rozerem. see ramelteon

schizoaffective disorder, 158
schizophrenia, 26, 37
    acute intervention, 48-51
    antipsychotic drug therapy,
        48-52, 80, 84, 86-88, 90,
        94-95, 97-98, 106, 112-13
    beta-blocker therapy, 215
    clinical course, 49
    diabetes risk, 62
    mood-stabilizing medications
        for, 159, 171
seasonal affective disorder, 153-54
second-generation antipsychotic
    medications, 20, 37-38,
        42-44, 71
    advantages, 47-48, 71
    effectiveness, 44-45
    injections, 108-9
    mechanism of action, 27, 40,
        41-42
    as mood-stabilizing medica-
        tions, 155-56
    side effects, 45-46, 47, 110-11
    see also antipsychotic medica-
        tions; aripiprazole; clozapine;
        olanzapine; paliperidone;
        quetiapine; risperidone; zip-
        rasidone
seizures, antipsychotic medication
    side effect, 69, 74-75
Seldane. see terfenadine
selective norepinephrine reuptake
    inhibitors, 136

borderline personality disorder
    treatment, 250
selective serotonin reuptake inhibi-
    tors, 21
    borderline personality disorder
        treatment, 250
    drug-drug interactions, 3, 175
    drug-drug interactions, 78,
        134-35, 148
    indications, 115, 117, 200
    mechanism of action, 127-28
    side effects, 132-34
    suicide risk, 126-27, 134
    use in pregnancy, 136
    withdrawal, 135-36
    see also antidepressant medica-
        tions; citalopram; fluoxetine
selegiline patch, 147, 251
Seroquel. see quetiapine
serotonin 2a receptor blockers, 21
serotonin and norepinephrine
    reuptake inhibitors, 21, 115,
        129-30
    drug-drug interactions, 134-35
    side effects, 132-34
    withdrawal, 135-36
    see also antidepressant medica-
        tions
serotonin and serotonergic system,
    24-25, 28, 40
    antidepressants with indirect
        action on, 137-39
serotonin blockers, 40-42
serotonin reuptake blockade, 22
serotonin syndrome, 3-4, 135
sertindole, 98
sertraline, 3-4, 129
Serzone. see nefazodone
sexual side effects
    antidepressant medications,
        133, 137, 138, 139, 144, 205
    antipsychotic medications, 40,
        47, 67, 79, 85
    treatment, 197

side effects
   compliance and, 13–14
   individual differences, 16
   initiating treatment, 15, 16
   significance of, 3
   see also specific class or type of
      medication; specific effect;
      specific medication
Sinquan. *see* doxepin
sleep apnea, 201
sleeping medications, 22–23,
      185–86
   antianxiety drugs and, 185–86
   antidepressant medications,
      137, 204–6
   antihistamines, 207
   benzodiazepines, 189, 191–92,
      202–3
   costs, 271
   GABA-A agonists, 203–4
   list of, 268–69
   melatonin-based, 206–7
   treatment decisions, 200–202
   types of, 202, 207–8
smoking
   cessation strategies, 23, 125,
      140, 237–38
   drug interactions, 33, 60, 78
social phobia, 124
sodium levels, 175
Sonata. *see* zaleplon
Stevens–Johnson syndrome, 174,
      178, 228–29
stimulant medications, 228
   for depression, 223–24
   for posttraumatic stress disor-
      der, 221–23
Strattera. *see* atomoxetine
Suboxone. *see* buprenorphine
substance abuse treatment, 23,
      232–38
   medication list, 269
substance use
   depression treatment and, 118

street drug–medication interac-
      tions, 60
suicidal behavior or ideation, anti-
      depressant medications and,
      126–27, 134
Symmetrel. *see* amantadine
synapse, 24

tardive dyskinesia, 40, 210
   antipsychotic medication side
      effects, 62–63, 65
   management, 65
   symptoms, 64–65
Tegretol. *see* carbamazepine
temazepam, 203
   indications, 185
Tenex. *see* guanfacine
Tenormin. *see* atenolol
terfenadine, 33
therapeutic relationship, 6–8, 239
   borderline personality disorder
      treatment, 245
   strategies to promote compli-
      ance, 12–14
thioridazine, 67, 103
thiothixanes, 21
thiothixene, 104
Thorazine. *see* chlorpromazine
thyroid dysfunction, lithium and,
      161–62
tiagabine, 183
Topamax. *see* topiramate
topiramate
   borderline personality disorder
      treatment, 249
   dosage, 182
   indications, 155, 181–82, 235
   side effects, 182, 235–36
traditional antipsychotics. *see*
      first-generation antipsychotic
      medications
tranylcypromine
   dosage, 145
   drug-drug interactions, 3–4

tranylcypromine (*continued*)
    see also monoamine oxidase
        inhibitors
trazodone, 137, 205
triazolam, 203
tricyclic antidepressants
    assessment for treatment with,
        141–42
    classification, 21–22
    clinical applications, 141, 205–6
    dosage, 142
    drug-drug interactions, 3, 142,
        171
    serum levels, 142
    side effects, 142–44
    withdrawal, 144–45
trihexphenidyl, 66, 211
Trileptal. *see* oxcarbazepine
Trilifon. *see* perphenazine
types of medications, 2–3
tyramine-containing foods, 146–47

Valium. *see* diazepam
valproate, 166–67
valproic acid
    dosage, 167–68
    drug-drug interactions, 170–71
    formulations, 166–67
    indications, 155, 167
    laboratory monitoring, 168, 170
    serum levels, 168
    side effects, 167, 169–70
    toxicity, 169
    use during pregnancy, 168–69
varenicline, 237–38
venlafaxine, 130–31, 200
verapamil, 183–84

violent outbursts, treatment of,
    215
vision and eye problems
    antipsychotic medication side
        effects, 66–67
    topiramate side effects, 182
Viskin. *see* pindolol
Vyvanse. *see* lisdexamfetamine

weight gain
    antidepressant medication side
        effect, 133, 144
    antipsychotic drug side effect,
        61, 73, 83–84, 89–90
Wellbutrin. *see* bupropion
withdrawal
    alcohol, 193
    antidepressant medications,
        120, 144–45
    benzodiazepine, 195–96

Xanax. *see* alprazalom

zaleplon, 204
ziprasidone, 51, 53, 54
    for acute mania of bipolar disor-
        der, 56
    borderline personality disorder
        treatment, 254
    dosing, 90–91
    formulations, 90
    indications, 90, 91
    side effects, 89–90, 91–93
Zoloft. *see* sertraline
zolpidem, 203–4
Zyban. *see* bupropion
Zyprexa. *see* olanzapine